T H I N S O F A S T

THIN
SO *FAST*

MICHAEL R. EADES, M.D.

WARNER BOOKS

A Warner Communications Company

Grateful acknowledgment is made for permission to reprint "Conversion Constants to Predict Body Fat—Women" and "Body Fat Percentages from the Penrose-Nelson-Fisher Equations," which appeared in A. Garth Fisher, *How to Lower Your Fat Thermostat*. Vitality House International, Inc. Used by permission.

Warner Books, Inc., 666 Fifth Avenue, New York, NY 10103

 A Warner Communications Company

Printed in the United States of America
First printing: February 1989
10 9 8 7 6 5 4 3 2 1
Library of Congress Catalog Card Number: 88-40616

Book design: H. Roberts

FOR
My wife, Mary Dan

Acknowledgments

First and foremost, I am indebted to Mary Dan Eades, M.D., my wife, colleague, and friend, for her inestimable help. Without her encouragement, grammatical skills, typing ability, medical knowledge, culinary talent, and capacity to endure me—a difficult person at best—this book would probably never have been written.

Cathy Hemming, my faithful agent, did a superb job of guiding me through the labyrinthine ways of the publishing world, gave encouragement and invaluable editorial assistance, provided the motivation needed now and then, delivered me from several dismal funks, and always showed me a good time on my visits to New York.

For much of the clarity of this book, thanks to Joann Davis, my editor at Warner. Her sometimes vexing habit of constantly wanting me to explain, clarify, and tie chapters together better has done nothing but make this a much better book. She was always available, returned all my calls, and was responsible for getting this project off the ground. As a first-time author, I couldn't have asked for a better editor.

To my sons, Ted, Daniel, and Scott, whom I love above all things, I offer thanks for their indulgence of an occasionally tyrannical father during the oftentimes stressful writing of this book. They endured with equanimity the inconvenience and upheaval this project has created.

I give many thanks to the long-suffering Dr. Stan Burns, who saw many of my patients in the clinic and shouldered much of the load so that I could have the time to devote to the writing of this book. Also, I am indebted to Michelle Hardy, Michelle Denton, Donna Harvey, and Carol Sitlington, who copied thousands of articles (by their estimate), fielded phone calls, and put up with and tried to accommodate my impossible demands. My capable assistant Carla Mathis deserves much praise for her good-natured ability to cope with the multitude of schedule changes and the appointment juggling my attention to this book required. Carla went above and beyond the call of duty in cheerfully taking on many of the onerous chores that I would otherwise have been obliged to perform. Kaye Easterling, Bobbie Via, Pat Slager—and the rest of my nursing staff— also deserve thanks for the help they rendered in accommodating my hectic schedule. And a word of thanks to Sheryll Ritchie for her help in the many projects that she undertook on my behalf to help gather data.

Thanks to my brother Dave, the business mind of our medical clinics, who attends to many of the niggling details that drive me crazy, and who shouldered much more of this burden while I was writing this book. And thanks to Susie Eades for always being willing to help with a multitude of tasks, usually on short notice.

I much appreciate the assistance given me by Earl Ramsey, Ph.D., and Jack Butler, university English professors and wordsmiths, who read and reread portions of this manuscript and provided invaluable advice on its improvement—some with which I agreed, some with which I didn't, but practically all of which I followed, deferring to their superior knowledge of the King's Ainglish.

A special word of thanks to Steve Boldt, the copyeditor on this project, whose superhuman effort in fixing this manuscript on very short notice made my life much easier.

Finally, I give thanks to James Pasley, Ph.D., Barry Sears, Ph.D., and others too numerous to mention, for their help in reading the manuscript and advising me on its improvement. Without their efforts, this would have been a much less complete book.

Author's Note:

I have no affiliation, financial or otherwise, with any of the companies whose products I discuss or recommend in this book, other than to purchase these products for my own use or for use in my practice.

The diet program I present in this volume is not identical with and should not be confused with Optifast, Medifast, HMR, or any of the other so-called Very Low Calorie Diets (VLCD). These VLCD typically contain 500 or fewer calories and should be undertaken *only* under the continuing supervision of a qualified physician. The dietary regimen described in *Thin So Fast*, although designed on the same physiological principles as these very low calorie protein-sparing fasts, will produce a slightly slower weight loss as a result of modifications I have made with the safety of the reader in mind. However, the *Thin So Fast* regimen, if followed properly, will bring about a safe, very rapid weight loss.

Contents

An Important Medical Note

Before beginning this or any other medical or nutritional regimen, consult your physician or other health care practitioner to be sure it is appropriate for you.

The information in this book reflects the author's experiences and is not intended to replace individualized medical advice. Any questions on symptoms, general or specific, should be addressed to your physician.

Introduction

*F*OR some time now, one of my hobbies has been collecting diet books. It started out, not as an idle pastime, but as a quest for the solution to my own weight problem. I kept hoping, just as every overweight person does, that the latest book would be the one that would work its dietary magic and solve the problem of my bulging waistline. I bought each new book as soon as it came out—never waiting for the paperback edition—and worked to overcome the biases engendered by my medical training so that I could believe each author's claims. I was promised, among other things, that I could "watch fat melt away," that I would "never be hungry again," that my pounds would "vanish," and even that I could "lose fat without dieting, hunger, or exercise!" Needless to say, none of these promised miracles occurred, and I relentlessly continued to pile on the weight—and add new books to my collection.

You will read in Chapter 1 how I finally lost all my excess weight by going on the protein-sparing modified fast. As everyone knows by now, this is the diet that enabled television talk-show hostess Oprah Winfrey to lose her sixty-seven pounds and fit, once again, into her Calvin Klein size 10 jeans. Ms. Winfrey went on the

Optifast program on which she consumed five protein shakes per day as her only form of sustenance while under the supervision of her physician. There are many such physician-supervised programs—Optifast, Medifast, R-Kane Products (Pro-Cal), Robard Corporation, Bariatrix International, Ultrafast, HMR, LifePlus, and several others. All these programs provide protein supplements that dieters consume instead of food, and all of them require physician supervision. The protein supplements come in a variety of forms— shakes (the most common), soups, gelatin desserts, puddings, hot chocolate, bouillons, fruit-flavor drinks, and in some cases cookies and other baked goods.

These programs differ from one another in the particular types of supplements (shakes vs. puddings vs. soups) used and in the protocol for taking them. All employ supplements that contain high-quality protein, more about which you will learn in Chapters 2 and 3. Most programs advocate that patients take these supplements exclusively instead of food, and as a result, they require close physician supervision to avoid problems. I have developed a modified version of these programs that is not as restricted and therefore much safer. I will give you the tools you need to undertake this program, which includes one meal per day along with four protein supplements, and which can be followed at home *after* you have discussed it with your physician.

At the same time that I started putting many of my patients on the supplemented fasting program, I began studying low-carbohydrate diets and their effects, and I developed the low-carbohydrate maintenance diet presented in Chapter 8. The low-carbohydrate diet has been around for many years; it isn't something I discovered (in fact, I have several books on the subject in my growing collection). But I developed a different method of counting carbohydrates that provides much more variety in a low-carbohydrate diet while at the same time increasing the amount of fiber present in what we eat (fiber inadequacy has been a criticism of low-carbohydrate diets).

As I continued my research on low-carbohydrate diets, my general medical practice gradually changed into one dealing exclusively with weight loss. I put my overweight patients first on the protein-sparing fast, and then on a low-carbohydrate maintenance diet. I monitored their blood values closely during their time with me, and I found that the claims made by the proponents of low-carbohydrate diets were indeed true—serum cholesterol and high blood pressure fall. I pored through medical journals trying to find out why.

What I discovered is that we live today in a "high-complex-carbohydrate" world in which fiber is on everyone's mind. We are constantly exhorted not only by the lay press but by the medical press as well to eat mainly fruits and vegetables—diets high in "complex carbohydrates." We are warned against the dangers of red meat and excess protein. Many "health-conscious" people would rather starve than eat an egg. Everyone is terrified of dietary cholesterol—a fact not lost on the food-processing industry. Today, many manufacturers produce products made of highly saturated plant oils and cover them with labels that shout "CHOLESTEROL FREE" or "CONTAINS NO CHOLESTEROL." As far as I am concerned, this verges on false advertising. Plants don't synthesize cholesterol, so they can't possibly contain cholesterol. But that doesn't mean these products are harmless. Often the saturated fats in these products are the culprits in elevating blood cholesterol, yet most consumers are distracted from this fact by the "contains no cholesterol" labeling.

So prevalent is the high-complex-carbohydrate, "eat mainly fruits and vegetables" mode of thinking, that many research scientists, physicians, and others who should know better are biased. They have bought into the notion that a diet high in complex carbohydrates is the ideal. And no matter how much the evidence might point in the other direction, they are resolute in their stance that we should all eat fruits, vegetables, and whole-grain breads almost to the exclusion of anything else. I have been to medical conferences where medical researchers have presented their findings, the conclusions of which scream out "low-carbohydrate diet," but they proceed to blithely state that these findings indicate that we should all stay on "high-complex-carbohydrate" diets.

A year ago I attended a seminar and heard a medical researcher present the evidence his group had obtained from a meticulously done, carefully controlled study. Their study correlated a high intake of carbohydrates with chronically elevated insulin levels, then correlated these high insulin levels with hypertension, elevated serum cholesterol, and obesity. After he made his presentation, he asked the question: "What does this tell us about how we should treat our patients with these problems?" It was obvious to me that a low-carbohydrate diet would do the job, but he answered his own question with "We should keep them on diets high in complex carbohydrates." I was stunned, but I soon got used to it; no matter what the evidence indicated, the conclusion was always the same —consume a diet rich in complex carbohydrates.

There are a few voices crying out in the wilderness in favor of fewer carbohydrates—Dr. Scott Grundy's group at the University of Texas, and Dr. Gerald Reaven's group at Stanford, to name a couple of the most vociferous. Both these researchers have published papers questioning the role of high-complex-carbohydrate diets in the treatment of non-insulin-dependent diabetes, but at this point at least, even they haven't come out for low-carbohydrate diets for the general overweight population.

As I gathered information and wrote protocol booklets for my patients who were on the low-carbohydrate diet, the idea of writing a book on the subject began to grow. I initially intended to write the definitive book on low-carbohydrate dieting, but I decided to incorporate my experience helping my patients reduce on the protein-sparing modified fast, since it is actually a low-carbohydrate/high-protein diet.

Once I made the decision to follow through on this book idea, I increased my efforts to expand my collection of diet books. Everywhere I went, I rooted through used-book stores and flea markets and found diet books of all ages. Almost all were examples of the type of book I did not want to write.

At my weight clinics in Arkansas I conduct weekly seminars for my patients, and I am amazed at how hungry they are for knowledge. They want to know why a specific regimen works the way it does. They are interested in the physiological and nutritional basis for all the recommendations I make concerning *their* health. (I believe that the decade of the nineties will be the decade in which Americans take charge of their own health instead of relying on various health care professionals to rescue them from their own excesses.) Based on the thirst for nutritional information exhibited by my patients (and I assume, the nation as a whole), and my knowledge of what I didn't want a diet book to be, I structured this book.

Most of the diet books in my collection make grandiose claims without any specific scientific basis to back up these claims. And I thought they addressed the reader in a condescending fashion as if he were a moron incapable of understanding anything other than trite phrases exhorting him to watch his "fat melt away." The book

I was in full end-of-the-year fat bloom, awaiting January 1st to start my annual diet. As we shook hands, my father, who has all the tact of a full-length mirror, commented that I looked "fat as a pig"! I laughed it off, of course, but the remark hit home and jarred me into facing the reality that I was carrying 215 pounds on a frame that carried 175 when I was in the best shape ever. At forty pounds overweight, I was, at least with respect to my diet, careening out of control. Something had to be done.

I had read in medical journals about a weight-loss program—the Protein-Sparing Modified Fast (or PSMF)—that was gaining acceptance among physicians across the country and being offered primarily through teaching hospitals. The PSMF had been developed in the early 1970s primarily at Harvard Medical School and Mt. Sinai Hospital in Cleveland as a method of treating extremely overweight individuals in a hospital setting. These researchers discovered a way to avoid the main problem—loss of muscle tissue—experienced in both total fasting and in extremely low-calorie diets: provide adequate protein intake and almost no carbohydrates. This regimen proved so successful in the hospital setting that it was eventually adapted to the clinical (outpatient) setting where results were excellent. In addition to rapid weight loss—most people lose from 2.5 to 5.3 pounds per week—dieters on the PSMF reported virtually no hunger while maintaining high levels of energy, and thanks to the regimen's simplicity, they had no food decisions to make or complicated menus to prepare. The PSMF regimen supplied all the required nutrients in the form of powdered protein supplements that the dieter reconstituted as a beverage and consumed either five times a day in lieu of food or four times a day with a single serving of meat and salad depending upon the protocol followed. These supplements were manufactured commercially but supplied to physicians only. I contacted one of the companies that produced the protein supplements, expressed my interest, and soon received their training-program literature. After studying the materials and reading all the cited medical studies, I was convinced that the regimen worked well and was safe, but—from the viewpoint of a man who had eaten three large meals a day plus snacks all his life—four protein shakes, a piece of meat, and a salad each day seemed a little draconian. At this point, however, I knew I needed help. I ordered the supplements and embarked on the program.

The results astounded me. I lost weight more rapidly than on any diet I had ever been on. After the first few days, I was never hungry, and I had an unbelievable amount of energy. In eight weeks, I dropped from 215 down to 178 pounds and felt uncommonly well the entire time. And best of all, the weight came off in all the right places. I didn't look gaunt as I had before after losing weight quickly, and I was able to wear clothing that I hadn't been able to get into for several years. (Isn't it funny that people almost never throw away clothes that are too small for them; they're always sure that someday, they will be able to wear them again.) I had reached my goal weight, but experience had taught me that the easy part was over. I had *lost* weight before—although never this easily—but the real trick was going to be in keeping it off, for as all dieters know, weight loss is a snap compared to maintenance.

I knew that the PSMF was basically a low-carbohydrate, high-protein diet in powdered supplement form, so I decided to put myself on a low-carbohydrate, high-protein diet in food form as my maintenance program. Low-carbohydrate diets are composed primarily of lean meats, cheeses, eggs, and other high-protein foods, while limiting the intake of starchy, sweet foods. This plan worked well for me, and I have been able to maintain my weight within a five-pound range since. My energy level has remained high, I get much more accomplished, and my serum cholesterol and triglycerides have dropped markedly.

Many of my regular patients who happened to be overweight observed my dramatic weight loss and became interested in trying the PSMF. I put several of them on the program, and all did well. These patients told others, and soon I had more patients coming to me to lose weight than patients who were suffering from other problems. I discovered that this new dimension I had added to my practice was both fulfilling and enjoyable. As the weight-loss portion of my practice increased almost exponentially, I made the decision to give up my general practice and have since limited my practice solely to the treatment of obesity.

I used the PSMF exclusively in the weight-loss phase of the program I was developing. My patients, most of whom consumed four protein shakes and one meal daily, had remarkable success in losing weight quickly, but once on maintenance they were not so fortunate. At first, I adhered to the standard practice of slowly weaning patients from the PSMF onto a low-calorie diet. Even though I was myself doing well on a low-carbohydrate, high-protein diet, I felt that it would be more prudent to treat my patients in a more medically conventional fashion. All the major PSMF programs around the country used a standard low-calorie regimen, and I saw no reason to do things differently. I saw no reason, that is, until I realized that almost all my patients were gaining their weight back after they went off the PSMF. After working diligently to lose excess weight, it is needless to say that it was frustrating for these patients—and for their physician—to begin almost immediately to gain it back. All concerned were distressed.

I decided that if the statistics were indeed true—and they certainly appeared to be in my practice—that ninety percent of patients were doomed to regain their weight, then our standard methods of treatment must be faulty. Or that a ten-percent success rate was all we could hope for. I knew that many virulent cancers had better successful treatment rates than that, and it seemed incredible to me that something as seemingly simple as being overweight could be so difficult to treat.

At a bariatrics conference (bariatrics is the medical specialty that deals with the treatment of obesity), one of the speakers, Dr. Peter Lindner, a well-respected authority, made the following statement concerning the ineffectual treatment methods we were all using: "If it doesn't work, change it!" Pondering this statement, I was prompted to consider seriously putting my patients on a low-carbohydrate, high-protein maintenance diet similar to the one I had found so effective for myself. It seemed absurd to me that we could have such a remarkable, effective tool as the PSMF to aid in the loss of weight, but nothing similar to aid in maintenance.

I initiated a survey among my patients to find what diets they had been successful with in the past. As might be expected, many of these patients had been on a multitude of diet plans and had a pretty good idea as to what had been most successful for them. To my surprise, most said that the best, easiest-to-follow diet, and the one that had worked most effectively, had been a low-carbohydrate diet. Still, these people were overweight, or they wouldn't have been in my office. So, although the low-carbohydrate diet—at least in the form tried by most of these patients—was not totally effective, it seemed like a good place to start. Upon questioning my patients about why they had abandoned this diet regimen, the most frequent complaint voiced was that it was limited and boring; most had tired of eating the same foods again and again. Some patients were also concerned about the safety of a diet that allowed the eating of unlimited amounts of red meat and fat. Although I knew that the diet I had been following, while high in red meats, eggs, and oils, had not raised my cholesterol or triglycerides—in fact quite the reverse—my personal case history was not enough upon which to build my maintenance diet.

I went to the university library and searched through the medical literature to find all the information I could on the effects of low-carbohydrate, high-protein diets, with the goal in mind to derive some modification of the regimens of the past that would provide more variety while at the same time being medically safe. The diet that I developed, with the help of my staff and patients, used in conjunction with the PSMF, is the basis for this book. As we proceed, I will address the safety issue, and you can determine for yourself how much variety is allowed.

Now I've told you my story, but what about others? What kinds of people go on the PSMF, and for what reasons? Most of my patients are from twenty-five to fifty or more pounds overweight, and many have medical problems as a result of their obesity. A number of them undertake the program strictly for convenience—no other diet is as simple. Let me introduce you to several patients from my practice and show you how the PSMF helped them.

PSMF Patients

Patricia L. is a typical example. She was 5'5" tall and thirty-seven years old when she came to see me because she had gradually embellished her medium frame until she weighed nearly two hundred pounds. Her ankles and knees hurt constantly due to the excess weight she carried, her blood pressure was elevated (her internist had cautioned her to lose weight two years earlier), and she was having frequent episodes of lower-back strain. What brought her to my office, however, was that her high school reunion was to take place the coming summer, and she wanted desperately to look the same as she did when she graduated twenty years earlier.

She told me that she had been "skinny as a rail" while growing up, and that her favorite foods were ice cream, hamburgers, pizza, and doughnuts, all washed down with soft drinks. She had eaten these foods without restraint yet had never gained a pound. In fact, she told me incredulously, she had even tried to gain weight to fill out her figure. Now, she laments, she eats salads, some vegetables, minuscule portions of meat—only lean—and drinks nothing but diet soft drinks, yet she continues to "pork up." She had tried several different "crash" diets, which had enabled her to lose some weight, which she had quickly regained. On more detailed questioning, she admitted to partying on weekends, and sure, she would "occasionally pig out" on potato chips, pastries, and other junk foods. "Doesn't everyone?"

Her family history is also typical. Her father, age sixty-three, has severe high blood pressure for which he takes three medications a day, and he had heart bypass surgery three years ago. He diets constantly in an effort to keep his cholesterol in check, and to keep his weight under two hundred pounds. (He weighed around two hundred sixty when he had the first episode of chest pain that led to his heart surgery). He, like his daughter, was very thin as a youth. Patricia's mother, age sixty-one, is obese, weighs almost one hundred eighty pounds, carries most of her excess fat on her hips, and has high blood pressure that she treats herself as the mood strikes her with prescription diuretics. She was also thin throughout adolescence but started to gain in her midtwenties. Patricia's siblings—all younger—are following the same pattern.

On physical exam, I found Patricia to have a moderately elevated blood pressure of 140/102, but except for her obesity, to be otherwise unremarkable. Apart from an elevated serum cholesterol and elevated serum triglycerides (a measure of fat in the blood), her lab results were within normal limits.

I discussed the PSMF with Patricia and warned her that it was not to be taken lightly. She was to follow it exactly as instructed, with no straying from the protocol. I asked her about the many times she had lost then regained weight in the past; why would the results be different this time? Would she regain after the reunion?

"Oh, I've learned my lesson," she assured me, "after I lose this time, I'll keep it off."

"I've learned my lesson"—that phrase, along with—"I don't know why I gain, I don't eat anything"—are the most often heard statements in a diet doctor's office. People seem to learn these same lessons multiple times.

Patricia apparently did learn her lesson. She lost sixty-seven pounds in eighteen weeks. She ended up with 22 percent body fat (low normal for her age) and a normal blood pressure, while the pain in her knees, ankles, and back vanished. Her elevated serum cholesterol and triglycerides returned to normal, and she reached her goal weight well before her reunion.

Patricia has managed to maintain her weight within a five-pound range for the past two years. She still occasionally "pigs out" on junk food, but she has learned how to recover from these binges with her figure intact. She has been the inspiration for many of her friends who have become my patients. Unfortunately, her parents remain unconvinced and continue to deteriorate physically.

Robert M. is a middle-aged accountant who travels during the week auditing businesses throughout Arkansas. He has slowly gained weight over the past fifteen years and was thirty-five pounds over his ideal weight when he came to see me. Robert's problem was that his travel schedule made it difficult to undertake a conventional diet; Monday through Friday, he ate every meal in a restaurant. Most restaurants in small towns in the South serve liberal portions of fried foods with potatoes, and cornbread or biscuits—meals that are high in both fat and carbohydrates, a disastrous combination for weight control.

The PSMF appealed to Robert mainly because of its simplicity; he carried his supplements with him and mixed them as needed. He felt better and was much more productive because he usually worked through lunch while sipping on a protein shake. His only gripe was that the supplements couldn't be put on his expense account as could his meals.

Robert lost thirty-five pounds in a little under two months. He worried that when he had to start eating restaurant food again, his weight would return. I assured him that if he followed the instructions I gave him on dealing with fast foods and dining out, he would successfully maintain his lower weight. It has been almost two years now since he completed the weight-loss phase of the diet, and he is still at his post-PSMF weight, despite eating daily at the same diners that put on his weight in the first place.

Sue M.'s history is a little different. She had always been slender until age thirty-three when her third child was born. She was unable to lose the final fifteen pounds after her pregnancy. Sue was an active person who threw herself into everything with great gusto, including her attempts to lose weight. She did all the things that had worked in the past: aerobics class, walking daily, and swimming, all while leading her normally active life. She even tried dieting for the first time in her life—unsuccessfully.

She presented herself at my office wanting to go on the PSMF. I told her that she could start after a thorough medical work-up, but that it seemed to me like an awfully expensive proposition to lose only fifteen pounds (the physical exam required includes an EKG and extensive laboratory evaluations, and it can be relatively costly per pound if only a few pounds need be lost). She was not to be deterred. It took her a month to lose the weight, and she has kept it off since. She now follows the low-carbohydrate, high-protein maintenance regimen with the same fervor and determination that she has for everything else she does.

As in my own case and those of Patricia, Robert, and Sue, patients who carefully adhere to the plan can expect to lose from 2.0 to 5.0 pounds per week, with almost all the loss coming from the body's fat stores. Remarkably, this loss takes place in the absence of any real hunger, and most people report increased energy levels and a feeling of euphoria. Probably the most often heard remark from patients on this program is, "This is the easiest diet I've ever been on."

If you are overweight, concerned about your cholesterol and blood pressure, and seem to drag through the day, then I suggest that you read this book carefully, have a thorough physical exam, and discuss the book with your doctor. Then, prepare to make a remarkable change in your life. Once you start the PSMF, you will see an amazing difference in the way you look and feel in a very short time.

Because the PSMF is so different from any other diet program you may have been on, it will be helpful to your understanding of it to see how the program was developed. Also, by knowing the intricacies of the regimen and how it works physiologically, I think you will be more inclined to adhere to the plan precisely as outlined in later chapters. First, we will see exactly how the PSMF works and the vast amount of research that went into its development.

2

The History of the Protein-Sparing Modified Fast

Total Fasting

Man has practiced fasting, either voluntarily or of necessity, since the dawn of his existence. Primitive man undoubtedly underwent many unwanted and unbargained-for fasts as a result of scarcity of game or drought. In fact, much of the trouble that modern man has with obesity is a genetic result of this feast-and-famine cycle—most people alive today are descendants of prehistoric ancestors who were able to efficiently store fat and survive the famines. Many religions include fasting as a part of their ritual beliefs, to cleanse the spirit, as a purification rite, a penance, or a sacrifice. More recently, in the 1920s and 1930s, faddists embraced fasting as a panacea for all ills. They claimed that it cleared the mind, increased endurance, and generally improved health. It wasn't until very recently that fasting was studied medically as a method for weight control.

In the late 1950s, several controlled studies were done in which very obese patients were hospitalized and put on total fasts under physician supervision. These studies were performed to determine if fasting was a viable method for weight control. No one doubted that total abstinence from food would bring about the loss of weight, but questions were raised about the safety of this approach. As these carefully monitored patients proceeded with their fast, it appeared as if all the claims of the faddists were indeed true. These patients reported that they were much more energetic, were never hungry, and in general had a feeling of great euphoria, while at the same time losing large amounts of weight. The laboratory studies and electrocardiograms, however, told a different story.

All of the patients were found to have severe fluid and mineral loss, metabolic acidosis, nitrogen loss (a sign of muscle breakdown), vitamin depletion, electrolyte imbalances, and hyperuricemia (elevated blood uric acid). Surprisingly, this disastrous internal picture was present in the face of a feeling of great well-being.

Let's briefly examine how and why these problems developed. On a true fast, people consume nothing but water. Since there is no carbohydrate intake, serum insulin levels fall, causing the kidneys to excrete sodium, potassium, and large amounts of fluid. As fat is broken down to provide energy, ketoacids (or ketone bodies) are produced that make the blood more acid, causing more fluid to be removed by the kidneys in an effort to correct the excess acidity. No vitamins or trace elements are taken in, yet the body continues to carry on the processes for which these nutrients are essential, leading to depletion. While the kidneys are busy excreting all the excess acid that is produced, they cannot adequately purge the body of uric acid (a protein-breakdown product), and oftentimes, severe attacks of gout are precipitated. Muscle, as well as fat, is being catabolized (utilized by the body for energy) and gotten rid of as nitrogenous waste. Unfortunately, not just skeletal muscle is catabolized, but heart muscle as well. As the potassium level falls, heart muscle becomes more excitable, and this, coupled with its weakened state, can lead to serious and even fatal rhythm disturbances. This doesn't sound like a healthy picture, does it? The amazing thing, however, is that all of these potentially devastating changes take place while the patient is blissfully unaware and is actually "feeling better than ever before." When you hear someone recommend a diet solely on the basis of how it makes you feel—remember this lesson.

How, you might ask, could one possibly feel well with all this potential for disaster developing? This effect has been attributed to the presence of the ketoacids or ketone bodies circulating in the blood, and their action on the central nervous system. The brain, which normally uses only glucose for energy, after a brief period of adaptation (usually two to three days), can employ ketone bodies for this purpose. It is thought that this altered energy utilization by the brain is responsible for the euphoria and lack of hunger experienced on a total fast.

Great amounts of weight are lost rapidly on a total fast, but as I have said before, not all from fat. In fact, almost one-half of the weight lost the first month, and one-third to one-fourth of the weight lost in subsequent months, is muscle tissue. Although big losses look great on the scales, when achieved by the loss of large amounts of muscle (which is very heavy tissue relative to fat), they are not permanent. When fasters resume eating, they invariably overcompensate in an effort to replace this lost lean-tissue mass and regain their weight very quickly.

The positive aspects of a total fast appeal very much to the person desperate to lose weight: rapid weight loss, little hunger, no need to prepare a special diet, and a feeling of euphoria. The potential problems, however, make a total fast a dangerous undertaking and an unacceptable means of weight reduction.

Modifying the Fast

In the 1970s, medical scientists at Harvard Medical School and Mt. Sinai Hospital in Cleveland took the first steps in the development of the protein-sparing modified fast when they began to search for methods by which the benefits of fasting could be maintained, while at the same time eliminating the dangers. Since most of the problems occurring in a full fast are the result of muscle wasting, potassium loss, and vitamin depletion, researchers looked first for ways to correct these hazards. Muscle is wasted because it is broken down to provide glucose (blood sugar) through a process called gluconeogenesis. In an attempt to arrest this process, researchers first provided a small amount of intravenous glucose to the fasting patients. They thought that perhaps by supplying glucose—the end product of muscle breakdown—to the tissues, the muscle would be spared. Surprisingly, the muscle wasting continued.

The next step was to try adding protein to the diet. It seemed reasonable to provide patients with a low-calorie protein supplement augmented with potassium and the necessary vitamins. With the addition of even small amounts of protein, the muscle wasting decreased strikingly. The first groups to study this method used protein in the absence of any carbohydrate, and they reported that patients experienced loss of hunger, increased energy levels, and euphoria. These patients had high levels of ketones in their blood, which were being eliminated via the urine and breath. There was some concern on the part of many researchers that these levels of ketosis (elevated blood ketones) could in some way be harmful. They then added a small amount of glucose to the protein formula to decrease this ketosis. The patients reported no diminishing of their feelings of well-being as their levels of ketosis dropped. They continued to lose weight, although not at the same rate as patients did on the total fast. The difference was that the weight lost was practically all fat with little muscle breakdown.

This slight loss of muscle tissue caused considerable concern to the researchers, who were attempting to completely arrest the wasting of lean-body mass. They increased the amount of protein in the supplement to higher and higher levels, hoping that a point would be reached where no muscle was lost, and patients would be in positive nitrogen balance, or at least in equilibrium. (Nitrogen is a component of protein and muscle that can be measured in urine. When the amount of nitrogen taken in by a person is greater than the amount eliminated as waste, the person is said to be in positive nitrogen balance, or is adding to his muscle mass. If excess nitrogen is lost, then muscle is being broken down.) Patients on this modified fast were never in positive nitrogen balance regardless of the amount of protein consumed. Finally, it was decided that this small muscle loss represented a decrease in muscle size due to lack of need rather than due to some failure of use of the protein supplement. As these very obese patients lost weight, they did not need as much muscle mass to support them. Just as body builders lose muscle mass when they stop lifting weights, these patients lost muscle mass as their weight diminished.

While patients were undergoing the modified fast, their health was rapidly improving in many ways. Their blood pressures dropped quickly, usually their blood cholesterol readings were much improved, they had better carbohydrate tolerance, and they reported significant relief of joint and spine pain. Interestingly, the dramatic blood pressure decreases seen in these patients were not due solely to their weight loss; their pressures dropped long before they had lost significant amounts of weight. In a later chapter, we will discuss the reasons for these changes in blood pressure readings and the importance of lowering your blood pressure.

All these studies described so far were performed with patients who were hospitalized throughout the duration of the research. As the protein supplements—at this stage basically egg albumin and a little glucose—were being refined as to varying amounts of protein and carbohydrate, doctors were realizing that the patients were experiencing no side effects of any magnitude, maintaining a fairly normal blood profile, and losing large amounts of weight rapidly. It seemed that all the virtues of fasting—rapid weight loss, in the absence of hunger—had been maintained, without the considerable dangers. The only drawback to the method was its enormous expense. Few overweight people could afford to be hospitalized for the several months necessary to lose substantial amounts of fat. The next step was to try this modified fast on obese subjects outside the hospital.

Outpatient Modified Fasting

In the 1970s, several research groups started outpatient modified-fasting programs—Drs. Genuth, Castro, and Vertes in 1974, Drs. Blackburn, Bistrian, and Flatt in 1975, and Drs. Howard and Baird in 1977. Patients were required to meet certain criteria before they were allowed to participate in the study. They had to weigh at least fifty pounds above their ideal body weight, be certain they were not pregnant, and have no serious health problems, including renal disease. People with high blood pressure and type II or adult-onset, non-insulin-dependent diabetes were accepted into the program; people with histories of recent heart attack, stroke, type I diabetes (insulin-dependent), and severe psychiatric disturbances were not. In the initial study, patients were hospitalized for the first week, then followed as outpatients with frequent returns to the clinic for weighing, counseling, and laboratory work. They were encouraged to continue their normal lifestyles, and to pursue their normal occupations.

The patients were started on a complicated regimen of supplementation in which glucose and a protein were taken from eight A.M. until midnight on an alternating basis at four-hour intervals. If these procedures seem overly precautionary to you, you must remember that when this study was done, this was all brand-new, and conceivably dangerous.

The physicians undertaking these outpatient studies anticipated that the patients would receive the same health benefits as those who participated in the hospitalization studies. They were concerned, however, about the potential for the patient's straying from the diet while not in the hospital. It is one thing to remain on a very limited diet while hospitalized and constantly monitored, but quite another to adhere while at home or work and being constantly tempted with a multitude of foods.

In most medical studies, standards are established at the outset that define what must be achieved for a regimen to be considered a therapeutic success. This study set two simple criteria for success: patients must stay on the program for a minimum of eight weeks *and* sustain a minimum weight loss of 2.2 pounds per week. The researchers hoped that the diet would result in a reduction in high blood pressure, carbohydrate intolerance, and joint pain, but these were not a part of their definition of success.

What happened? Over two-thirds of the patients admitted to the program achieved success by the above criteria. Most of the one-third that failed lost the required amount of weight, but for a number of reasons they were not able to stay in the program for the required eight weeks. What about improvement in the above-mentioned medical problems? Let's read from the original research paper by Drs. Genuth, Castro, and Vertes as it was published in the November 18, 1974 issue of the *Journal of the American Medical Association*:

> Beneficial effects [of this regimen] included reduction in blood pressure of hypertensive patients, improvement in carbohydrate tolerance with discontinuation of insulin therapy in two diabetic patients, improvement in dyspnea [difficulty breathing] especially noted in patients with complicating pulmonary or cardiac disease, relief of back pain or joint pain, and decided increase in exercise tolerance and agility. Most patients expressed gratification at their perception of a better psychosocial status. Several did react adversely to their newly thinned state, unmarried women occasionally exhibiting panic at their enhanced attractiveness to men. . . . No major disability was noted even up to one year.

The success of this research inspired a succession of studies by this same group of investigators as well as others. The protocols changed as doctors became more comfortable with using the modified fast. It was no longer necessary for patients to be hospitalized even for the first week, and supplements were developed that were much more palatable while at the same time containing more nutrients. Many, many more patients were started on the modified fast, which was now being called the protein-sparing modified fast—"protein-sparing" because the patient's lean-body mass or protein was spared from being broken down, a "modified" fast because the patients were consuming supplements instead of going without any oral intake, but yet a fast because no "real" food was being eaten.

As the number of successful patients grew, the number of research hospitals offering the PSMF increased. It became possible in the early 1980s for overweight people living in most large cities to find a medical center that would accept them as patients, provide them with supplements, and monitor them on the PSMF. There was such demand for the program that facilities providing it were overrun with patients, and unfortunately, long waiting lists were soon the norm everywhere. Patients with serious medical problems as a result of their obesity were placed at the head of the line, and those patients merely overweight were often never gotten to. Most programs would not accept people who were not at least fifty pounds overweight. People who were only thirty-five to forty pounds overweight in some cases actually gained weight so that they would be accepted into a PSMF program.

As a result of this explosion of demand, several manufacturers developed supplemented fasting programs, and produced palatable, easily mixed supplements that are the standard today. The companies also developed formal training programs and standard protocols for physicians nationwide who wished to administer the PSMF. Consequently, many physicians in private practice (myself included) started treating patients with the PSMF using the protein supplements provided by these companies. Subsequently, many other manufacturers have developed similar products for marketing to physicians, and currently, thousands of physicians are using the PSMF as a part of their practice. This increased number of physicians trained to administer the PSMF has created a place in which those patients with fewer than fifty pounds to lose may participate in a supervised fasting program. In fact, since the first physician-supervised programs started, several hundred thousand people have lost weight quickly and without significant medical problems using the protein-sparing modified fast.

The expense of participating weekly in a physician-supervised fasting program may be prohibitive for some, and for otherwise healthy patients may not be necessary. (Certain medical conditions, however, necessitate that you remain under a physician's care while dieting; I have listed and discussed these in Chapter 5.) In this book, I am going to show you how you can safely and simply use the PSMF at home, and how to prepare your own protein supplements from a simple recipe (given in Chapter 6) that uses readily available, inexpensive ingredients. But let me stress the point once again that you should *not* begin this program until you and your physician have discussed it, you have undergone a complete physical examination with the specified laboratory studies, and you are certain that you do not suffer from any of the conditions that preclude your safe use of this kind of diet. Let me now tell you why.

Liquid Protein Disaster

Despite the enviable safety record of the PSMF, there have been some dark days in the history of modified fasting that we should review. Many of you may recall that there were some severe problems about ten years ago with the use of "liquid protein" diets for weight loss. In 1976, a book entitled *The Last Chance Diet* by Dr. Robert Linn and Sandra Lee Stuart was published advocating the use of what the author called a protein-sparing fast for rapid weight loss. Unfortunately, the supplements the author recommended were of poor quality protein and did not provide the necessary protein building blocks for maintaining lean-body mass. Patients took the supplements as they would medicine, a couple of tablespoonfuls at a time throughout the day. Since there were no carbohydrates in these supplements, patients rapidly developed a high level of ketosis, which, you remember, causes a sense of well-being. Dieters felt great and lost very large amounts of weight; unfortunately, some also lost their lives.

The medical literature documented that sixty people died while on this "protein-sparing" regimen, but physicians speculated that there were probably many more who died that were misreported. Most of these deaths were as a result of ventricular arrhythmias (aberrant heart rhythms) that were unresponsive to treatment, and that finally led to cessation of normal heart pumping, then death. Autopsy showed that the victim's heart muscle was damaged, probably from chronic protein malnutrition. Surprisingly, many of the patients who died were females between the ages of twenty-seven and thirty-five, who were previously, other than being overweight, in good health.

A review of the medical papers concerning these deaths revealed several interesting statistics. First, all deaths occurred in persons who had been on this regimen for two months or longer. Second, almost two-thirds of the patients had some underlying medical disorder that possibly contributed to their demise. About one-half of the patients were under medical supervision while on this regimen, and they were found to have normal electrocardiograms prior to starting the diet. Finally, most patients were found not to have hypokalemia (decreased levels of potassium in the blood that oftentimes cause arrhythmias). Researchers were unable to identify any particular patient profile that would identify seemingly normal persons who were at risk for undertaking a liquid protein diet.

I don't intend to frighten you with this information, but there are important facts we can learn from an analysis of these somber statistics. They are:

1. Stringent dietary regimens should not be undertaken lightly, as serious consequences sometimes result. The program described in the book you are reading has been developed with your safety in mind, so *do not* modify it.

2. Even on an inferior source of protein (which I absolutely discourage), serious consequences are unlikely to occur on a protein-sparing fast if patients remain on the regimen for no longer than two months. (Many patients have remained on the PSMF using a high-quality, complete protein for over one year without problems.)

3. Medical supervision is no guarantee of immunity from problems on a liquid protein diet. Don't misunderstand this point; I strongly recommend medical supervision for *any* exacting dietary regimen, but the record shows that on the old "liquid protein" diets several people died while being monitored.

4. It *is* possible to identify persons who have obvious medical problems that eliminate them as candidates for a similar program, but few criteria exist for identifying "normal" subjects who are at risk.

After evaluation of this information, the conclusion you should reach seems pretty obvious: don't attempt a liquid protein diet. Now, you may ask, if the PSMF as practiced by physicians everywhere, and as presented in this book, is based on supplements that are (1) liquid and (2) protein, is it not just "liquid protein" under another name? A very good question. Technically, because of their nature, the PSMF supplements can't be anything other than "liquid protein" (some of the newer commercial supplements are in cookie or cake form, but that is splitting hairs); however, the old "liquid protein diets" as described in the medical literature used a poor quality protein that was taken by the tablespoon as medicine rather than enjoyed as a food. In short, the "liquid protein diets" were little different from a total fast. As advocated in my regimen, and as practiced everywhere now, the PSMF supplements are a high quality protein and are taken in combination with a complete regimen of vitamins and minerals. They are fairly tasty—no one mistakes them for French cuisine—but the supplements aren't tossed back like cough medicine. Properly followed, the PSMF is extremely safe, and with the modifications made and detailed in this book, it is even safer. But the safety hinges upon using a *complete*, high quality protein in the preparation of the supplement powder, and in having a basic understanding of the nutrition and science involved. In the next chapter you will begin to acquire such knowledge as we plunge into an in-depth discussion of the basic nutritional precepts that I will be referring to throughout this book.

As we go through this book, chapter by chapter, you will see the evidence begin to mount that the PSMF is the most effective way currently available to lose large amounts of body fat quickly *and* safely.

3

Everything You Ever Wanted to Know About Nutrition . . . and Probably More

YESTERDAY'S dieters were content to be told what to do, and many—myself included—blindly followed the latest fad diet without regard to possible adverse health consequences; if the dieter lost weight, the diet was considered to be a success. This is not the case with today's much more health-conscious dieter. From the questions I field during weight-loss seminars in my clinic, it is obvious to me that the health aspects of any dietary plan are of primary importance to its followers. Gone are the days—thank God—when most people would unquestioningly accept any bizarre weight-loss scheme as long as sticking with it resulted in the promised loss of pounds. Now, people are concerned with the scientific underpinnings of not only diets, but even medical treatment regimens as well. They want to know what the side effects are, what possible drug interactions may occur, and what the long-term effects on their health might be.

Both the PSMF, since it requires a radical departure from standard dieting behavior, and the low-carbohydrate maintenance program I use, seemingly contrary to the current high complex-carbohydrate "wisdom," stimulate many thoughtful questions from people contemplating starting the program. At this point, you probably have most of the same questions my new patients do:

"What will happen to my cholesterol if I go on this diet and your maintenance plan?"

"I thought eating meat was bad for me?"

"I've heard that low-carbohydrate diets are not good for people. Doesn't your body need carbohydrates to function?"

"Aren't low-carbohydrate diets the same as high-fat diets?"

"What about fiber? Is there fiber in the protein supplements?"

"I've heard that there is very little fiber in low-carbohydrate diets, is that true?"

"Can you really get everything you need in these protein shakes and one meal and nothing else?"

Until you get the answers to these and many other questions, you may be a little reluctant to embark upon the PSMF wholeheartedly. I'm glad you asked these questions and this book will answer them. My purpose is not only to give you specific instructions on undertaking the entire regimen, but to provide you with the scientific rationale for why it works and why it will improve your health while it improves your figure.

You may, however, be eager to start losing weight and may not really want to plow through all the science at this point. After all, you don't have to know how to build a car in order to drive one successfully. *If this is your situation, you have my permission to charge ahead to Chapter 4, calculate your percentage of body fat, and then proceed on to Chapters 5 and 6, the real heart of the PSMF portion of the program, and get started.* If you do this, you must follow the instructions to the letter, and prepare your supplements using *only* the products I have listed. *Read Chapters 5 and 6 in their entirety before you start the diet.* After you are cruising along on the PSMF, please come back to this chapter and read it carefully at your leisure—then you will better understand the discussion of the maintenance program that you will begin as soon as you have achieved your goal weight. For those of you who wish to plunge ahead into the nutrition lesson now, let's begin.

Nutrition 101

To fully understand the workings of the PSMF and the low-carbohydrate maintenance diet, you must have a fundamental knowledge of the basic food groups and how your body uses them. When I say basic food groups, I don't mean breads and grains, dairy products, meats and fish, and fruits and vegetables—the famous "four basic food groups," but rather the three main groups into which all foods fall—*protein, carbohydrate,* and *fat.*

Since an understanding of what these main groups really are is essential to your understanding of how the PSMF works and why it is different from other diets, let me begin our discussion with these basic components. We will delve into these topics in some detail and then touch more briefly on vitamins, minerals, and electrolytes. After you are familiar with these subjects, we will use them as a basis to compare the PSMF and a low-carbohydrate diet with the typical American diet. Let's begin with protein—the most important component of the PSMF.

Protein

Protein is absolutely indispensable for life. All growth, tissue repair and regeneration, and recovery from infection, requires large quantities of protein, our most vital nutrient. If I were to ask you to name a part of the body that is made of protein, you would probably say muscle, and you would be correct. Protein does form muscle tissue, but it is also the major structural component of hair, ligaments, skin, and fingernails. It forms saliva, all enzymes (such as digestive enzymes), many blood components, immune cells, and the framework of our bones.

Protein molecules are made of groups of basic subunits called *amino acids,* which our bodies combine in various arrangements. The type of protein made depends upon which of the twenty-two different amino acids are used and how they are hooked together: it is a process controlled by our genes. In order to manufacture the proteins we need to live, we must provide our bodies with an adequate supply of these amino acids in the diet. The protein-manufacturing machinery of our bodies—the cells—can make some amino acids by rearranging the structure of other amino acids, but there are certain amino acids—the nine so-called *essential* amino acids—that the body cannot make, and these must be present in the diet for continued good health.

It is imperative that these essential amino acids not only be present, but be present in the proper proportions. A dietary shortage of one of the nonessential amino acids does not create a problem since the body can manufacture these by rearrangement of others.

If, however, a dietary shortage of even one of the essential nine amino acids occurs, no protein requiring it can be made. In other words, absolute quantity of dietary intake is not the issue; we can eat a pound of protein, but if it is incomplete by even one essential amino acid, it does us no good.

To help illustrate this important concept, let's say we are trying to build a brick wall—in this case, the brick wall represents a protein the body must synthesize. To build the wall, we will need to mix water and sand together with cement to form grout, which we spread between the bricks to "glue" them in place—so the basic components of wall-building are bricks, sand, cement, and water. We will let the cement represent one of the nine essential amino acids, so that we can see how varying its amount can affect the construction of the finished product: the completed protein or the brick wall. If we have adequate supplies of all components on hand, our wall is built without any problem; if we have more than adequate supplies of everything needed, we can build the wall and have materials left over which we can dispose of. (Our bodies do exactly this, getting rid of excess amino acids in the urine.) But if we have very little cement, it makes no difference that we may have a ton of bricks, a mountain of sand, and a river at our disposal—we can still only build a tiny portion of our wall. The deficiency of cement—a single necessary component—has prevented us from doing the job. The fact that we have many leftover bricks and a big pile of sand is of no consequence. The leftovers are wasted. So it is with incomplete protein: all essential amino acids must be provided or no protein can be built. The protein we eat must therefore be *complete*.

What Constitutes a Complete Protein?

Dietary protein is rated based upon the amounts of the various amino acids of which it is made. A protein source that has an amino acid profile similar to that required for making body tissues is called *high biological grade* protein; one deficient in a particular amino acid(s) would be termed *low biological grade* protein. Just as in the analogy of the wall, we can eat a huge amount of low quality protein and not be able to make as much usable body protein as from a small amount of high quality protein. On a typical, full-food diet, we generally are able to eat sufficient amounts of good quality protein without giving it much thought. A tuna sandwich, a chicken breast, a hard-boiled egg—all provide a fair amount of high bio-logical quality protein. Problems arise, however, when we try to formulate protein supplements for the PSMF, or when we go on very low-calorie or vegetarian diets. I cannot stress strongly enough how important it is that a high biological grade protein be used in the PSMF, so that problems related to protein deficiency discussed in the previous chapter do not arise.

We must consume adequate protein on a regular basis, because unlike carbohydrates and fats, protein cannot be stored in the body. Once we digest protein, it is used by the body to make new protein with any surplus eliminated in the urine. For this reason, people with poor kidney function have a difficult time eliminating the protein-breakdown products and must restrict their protein intake to a low—but still *adequate*—level. Most of us, however, have no difficulty in this regard if we drink enough fluid to make the amount of urine necessary to get rid of the excess. This is the reason I insist that you drink large quantities of water or other fluids once you start the PSMF or other high-protein diets.

What foods contain large amounts of good quality protein? Beef, pork, chicken, turkey, fish, dairy products, and eggs are all excellent sources of high biological grade protein. Most plants con-tain some protein, but they are often deficient in one or more es-sential amino acids. Some plants—such as soybeans, certain rices, oats, sunflower and sesame seeds—are good sources of protein, but usually not as good as meat, eggs, and dairy products. Vegetarians need to be careful to "balance" proteins from plant sources (eating one vegetable deficient in a particular amino acid along with one rich in it, but perhaps deficient in some other one), so that the net result is that all nine essential amino acids are present. Whatever the source—whether meat and eggs, balanced plant proteins, or high quality protein supplements—we must be certain to consume ample protein.

Fat

Fat is today's dietary villain, accused of causing heart disease, cancer, obesity, and a host of other maladies. We are conditioned in America to believe that if all fat were removed from our diet, we would live longer and be healthier. This belief is misguided, how-ever. Certain types of fat are as essential for life and health as protein.

The importance of fat has never been stated more eloquently than by Horace Davenport, Ph.D., D.Sc., author of *Physiology of the Digestive Tract*, a textbook used in many medical schools. Dr. Davenport says of fat: it is a "major structural component of the body. Because fat is insoluble in water, fat forms the membranes of cells and cell organelles; without fat the body would thaw and resolve itself into a dew."

Lipids—the medical term that encompasses all fats—like proteins, perform many vital functions in our bodies. Storage or depot fat—the kind that we have in overabundance when we are obese—acts both as a thermal blanket that insulates us from heat loss, and as a protective cushion for most tissues and organs. Lipids also constitute the basic structure from which sex hormones, steroid hormones, prostaglandins, vitamin D, and other vital substances are synthesized. Lipids are a readily available source of energy—one pound of body fat contains enough energy to allow a person to walk about thirty-five miles. (The amount of fat on a person weighing 150 pounds theoretically provides enough energy for that person to walk from St. Louis to Washington, D.C.) Cholesterol, more of a waxy substance than a fat, but a lipid nevertheless, forms an integral part of all cell membranes, makes the lining for nerves, and is present in large amounts in brain tissue. Cholesterol has also been implicated as a factor in coronary artery disease, and as a result, many people are concerned about the level of cholesterol in their blood. In Chapter 10, we will discuss in detail the role dietary cholesterol plays in the development of elevated serum cholesterol and the ways that the PSMF and other low-carbohydrate diets work to reduce serum cholesterol.

Dietary lipids can be divided into two categories based on consistency—fats and oils. Fats are solid or firm at room temperature, while oils can be poured. Most dietary lipid of animal origin—lard, bacon, etc.—is solid and therefore considered a fat, whereas lipid of plant origin is almost always liquid and therefore considered an oil. All fats and oils, like proteins, are composed of varying amounts of smaller subunits called *fatty acids*. Most oils and fats are not made of just one fatty acid, but are a combination of several, and the properties that are unique to olive oil, lard, butter, or any other fat or oil are dependent upon these specific combinations of the particular fatty acids that they comprise. The various fatty acids have their own distinct properties that are a function of the size of the fatty acid and whether it is saturated or unsaturated, and to what degree. The terms "saturated" fat and "polyunsaturated" fat are commonly used, but what do they really mean?

Saturated vs. Unsaturated Fat

Fatty acids are made of a chain of carbon atoms that are chemically hooked or bonded together to form the backbone of the molecule. The difference between saturated and unsaturated fats lies in the character of the bonds between these carbon atoms—whether the bonds are single or double. Chains that have all carbons connected with single carbon-to-carbon bonds can attach to the maximum number of hydrogen atoms and are said to be "saturated" with hydrogen. Chains with double carbon bonds cannot attach to as many hydrogens and are therefore "unsaturated" with hydrogen. The degree of unsaturation is determined by how many double bonds there are in the carbon chain—if only one double bond is present, the fatty acid is said to be *mono*unsaturated, but if two or more double bonds are in the chain, it is termed *poly*unsaturated. The single carbon-carbon bonds are much more stable than the double bonds, which means that the more unsaturated a fatty acid is, the more unstable it is. This variation in stability as a function of unsaturatedness is what causes the different actions of various fats in the body.

Oils and fats such as olive oil, corn oil, safflower oil, lard, and all the others are composed of a mixture of saturated, monounsaturated, and various polyunsaturated fatty acids. When you see an oil referred to as being polyunsaturated, it means that the fatty acids making up the bulk of the oil are predominately polyunsaturated, but both saturated and monounsaturated fatty acids are present as well. For example, safflower oil—considered by many a totally polyunsaturated oil—contains about 75 percent polyunsaturated, 14 percent monounsaturated, and even 10 percent saturated fatty acids. On the other hand, lard—thought by most to be a very saturated fat—contains approximately 14 percent polyunsaturated, 46 percent monounsaturated, and only 40 percent saturated fatty acids. When you buy corn oil (or any other oil or fat) at the supermarket, what you get is not some special distilled essence of corn with unique properties, but an oil with a specific combination of the three basic types of fatty acids—saturated, monounsaturated, and polyunsaturated—that are common to all oils and fats.

Since the carbon-carbon double bonds are unstable and easily broken, the more unsaturated a fatty acid is, the more unstable it is. Monounsaturated fatty acids are more stable than polyunsaturated fatty acids, and saturated fatty acids, since they contain no double bonds, are the most stable of all. Consequently, oils composed of primarily polyunsaturated fatty acids are relatively unstable. Our bodies are better able to break the weak double bonds of polyunsaturated fatty acids and form new substances from the resultant shorter carbon chains. Some of these products of polyunsaturated fatty acid breakdown—certain prostaglandins, for example—provide health benefits and are one of the reasons that polyunsaturated fats are good for us.

Monounsaturated fats such as olive oil and canola (rapeseed) oil are the subjects of much recent research that has linked the consumption of these oils with a decreased incidence of high blood pressure, heart disease, and elevated blood cholesterol. Many medical researchers believe that the low rates of heart attack and coronary artery disease found in Mediterranean countries may be attributed in part to the large consumption of olive oil common in that area.

Saturated fats—those thought to be harmful when consumed to excess—are found in high concentrations in domesticated animal meat, dairy products, and in certain plant oils. Most people are aware that fat of animal origin is highly saturated, but what about the plant oils? Aren't plant oils mainly unsaturated? Most are, but the tropical plant oils—palm oil, palm kernel oil, and coconut oil—contain much higher levels of saturated fats than lard and other animal sources of fat. Food manufacturers are turning more and more to these tropical oils instead of the more unsaturated vegetable oils for two reasons: (1) tropical oils have a longer shelf life, and (2) they are much easier to process. Let's digress here briefly and examine food processing operations as they relate to the various oils.

The relatively weak double bonds that give unsaturated oils the properties we discussed above also make these oils unstable when exposed to heat and light—the more unsaturated the oil, the more unstable. Oxygen molecules in the air attack these double bonds and produce a chemical reaction called oxidation that causes the oil to become rancid. Since rancid oil is neither a major seller at supermarkets, nor a big hit at the dinner table, food technologists were summoned to develop methods to prevent the oxidation process from taking place. The technique they developed, which is now used by most food processors, involves breaking some or all of the double bonds and forcing hydrogen atoms onto the carbon chain in a process called, logically enough, hydrogenation. After hydrogenation, the formerly polyunsaturated oil becomes "hydrogenated," or "partially hydrogenated"—the latter if not all the double bonds are destroyed; the oil becomes less prone to rancidity and has a longer shelf life. In short, it becomes a saturated fat, or at best, a less unsaturated fat.

If the end result of hydrogenation is the production of a saturated fat, why not just start with a saturated fat and not go through all the hassle? There are a couple of reasons. First, over the past twenty years most people have been conditioned to seek out polyunsaturated oils and avoid saturated fats. Second, these same people have been exhorted to decrease their consumption of cholesterol, and so they seek food products that contain little or none. Saturated fats of animal origin such as lard or butter contain varying amounts of cholesterol, but oils of plant origin, no matter how saturated they may be, contain *no* cholesterol. Unlike animals, plants don't require cholesterol for life, and therefore they don't synthesize it. As a result, plant oils never contain cholesterol. In an effort to satisfy the consumer demand for oils that are low both in saturated fat and in cholesterol content, food manufacturers have turned to these cholesterol-free oils of plant origin that are usually polyunsaturated and seem to fit the bill nicely. The manufacturers can, by applying varying degrees of hydrogenation, produce an oil product that has a longer shelf life, remains cholesterol free, and has the desired consistency—liquid or solid. These consumers purchase a "corn oil" margarine—most know that corn oil is predominantly polyunsaturated—not realizing that it has been hydrogenated to some extent (or not understanding what hydrogenation means), and they get a product that is probably as saturated as butter—but cholesterol free. How do the tropical oils mentioned above fit into this hydrogenation scheme?

The tropical oils are naturally so saturated that they don't require much, if any, hydrogenation to increase their shelf life, making them less expensive to produce. They are finding their way into more and more processed foods, being hidden or downplayed by the use of clever labeling designed to hide the amount of saturated fat. Since these oils are plant products, their cholesterol-free nature is prominently proclaimed on the package label, directing attention away from the degree of saturation of the oil. Sometimes the labels state that the product contains "one or more of the following: palm, palm kernel, cottonseed, peanut, soybean, safflower oil." But how much of which ones? Who knows. Unsuspecting buyers who would never consider eating lard get a product that is touted as cholesterol-free and presumably "healthful." They never realize that they are consuming much more saturated fat in these vaguely labeled products than in products made with the rendered animal fat they so disdain. I don't want to engage at this point in a diatribe against the mislabeling of foods, but I do want to make clear that there are sources of saturated fat other than of animal origin. But does it really matter; is the consumption of saturated fats unhealthful?

Saturated Fats and Health

Fats contribute much to the texture and palatability of foods, and without them, our diets would be bland. Much of what we consider "good" or "tasty" in foods comes from fat, and often from saturated fat. If we try to eliminate or severely restrict the amount of fat in the foods we eat, we will end up with a diet that is tasteless and too unpalatable to adhere to for any length of time. The greater the sacrifice we make in our diet, the less likely we are to stick with it unless there are overpowering health reasons to keep us on the more stringent regimen. In view of this fact, it seems reasonable to take a close look at the merits of a reduced-fat diet.

Most recent studies indicate that elevated levels of blood cholesterol correlate with an increased incidence of heart disease, but does an increased intake of cholesterol and/or other saturated fat cause an increase in the level of blood cholesterol? We will address this question in great detail in Chapter 10, but for now let me state that there is no unequivocal proof that increased consumption *of cholesterol alone* causes increased levels of blood cholesterol. Some studies have shown a correlation, but an equal number have shown none. This is an area of medicine that is currently embroiled in a great deal of controversy, with each side of the issue having its well-respected champion and long list of confirming research reports. It is safe to say now that there is no beyond-the-shadow-of-a-doubt proof on the cholesterol-consumption/blood-cholesterol-level issue.

Many researchers have shown that increases in blood cholesterol levels can be produced in *most* individuals by the addition of large amounts of saturated fat to their baseline diet. The operative word here is *addition;* nothing else in the diet is changed. Most of these studies are done by putting subjects on a restricted fat diet for a period of time and then measuring the levels of cholesterol in their blood. The researchers then add an increased amount of saturated fat to this diet in order to make it correspond in fat content to the typical American diet—or whichever diet they wish to compare— and then again measure the blood cholesterol. Usually, researchers find that the cholesterol levels rise after the addition of saturated fat to the diet.

If, however, instead of *adding* the saturated fat to the baseline diet, researchers *replace* a corresponding amount of carbohydrate with fat, these rises in blood cholesterol are generally not seen. In fact, the opposite often happens, and the blood cholesterol levels actually *fall.* Therefore, the elevation or decrease in levels of blood cholesterol resulting from saturated-fat consumption is also greatly dependent upon the level of carbohydrates a person ingests—a fact we will discuss in great detail as this book progresses.

Aside from matters of taste, how much fat do we require in our diets? And what kinds? Just as there are certain essential amino acids that must be obtained from the diet, are there corresponding essential fatty acids?

Are Specific Fats Essential?

There are three basic polyunsaturated fatty acids that are nec-essary for our well-being—linoleic, linolenic, and arachidonic acid. Scientists once thought that all three had to be obtained in the diet, but now we know that both linolenic acid and arachidonic acid can be synthesized from linoleic acid, making *linoleic acid* the only truly *essential fatty acid.* Fortunately, linoleic acid is present in large amounts in most vegetable oils, and in smaller amounts in most other fats, so that any diet containing these substances provides enough linoleic acid to prevent deficiency. But even though linoleic acid is the only absolutely essential fatty acid, evidence is mounting that we may obtain health benefits from eating several other kinds of fatty acids as well. In Chapter 10, we will examine the effects of these different fatty acids on the incidence of heart disease, high blood pressure, elevated cholesterol levels, and other medical conditions.

Carbohydrates

Carbohydrates are sugars, starches, and most fiber. Sugars and starches are readily available, inexpensive, and palatable, and they comprise from 40 to 60 percent of the typical American's diet. Carbohydrates are found in varying concentrations in all fruits, vegetables, grains, most dairy products, and in some shellfish. We are constantly urged to get most of our calories in the form of ever larger amounts of complex carbohydrates (starches and fibers), while reducing our intake of calories provided by fat and protein. As in the case with fats and protein, are certain carbohydrates essential? Let's turn again to Professor Davenport in *Physiology of the Digestive Tract*. He states that "dietary carbohydrate is entirely dispensable; nevertheless it is 50%–60% of the American mixed diet, and in many countries is a larger percentage." It has always seemed a little odd to me that we are exhorted to make a larger and larger portion of our diet carbohydrate—an entirely inessential nutrient—and to reduce, or replace, the foods—protein and fat—that are essential.

Carbohydrates—although found in a mixed state in most plant foods—can be divided into three basic categories: simple sugars, starches or complex carbohydrates, and fiber. Simple sugars are carbohydrates that require little digestion or enzymatic degradation to be converted to their ultimate destiny—blood glucose. Sucrose (table sugar), fructose (fruit sugar), and lactose (milk sugar) are some—but by no means all—of the simple sugars. (Some of these sugars are combinations of simple sugars—sucrose, for example, is a combination of one glucose molecule attached to one fructose molecule—and in the strictest scientific definition are not simple sugars. For the purposes of this book, however, we will define simple sugars to be single sugars or combinations of very few single sugars, while starches are combinations of many single-sugar molecules.) These sugars pass quickly through the digestive process and are rapidly converted to glucose—another simple sugar—which circulates in the blood and provides energy to certain tissues of the body—notably, the brain. Glucose is essential to our survival, but unlike protein and fat, both of which must be provided in the diet, it can be manufactured in the body. It can be synthesized quite easily from both protein and fat, and in turn, excess glucose can be converted into fat and into the nonessential amino acids. Since no dietary carbohydrate is required for the internal production of glucose, humans can consume diets totally deficient in carbohydrates and survive nicely. In fact, most prehistoric societies lived very well on diets almost devoid of carbohydrates—especially simple sugars. Today, Eskimos and other isolated groups continue to live lives free of heart disease and many other diseases of modern civilization on these same low-carbohydrate diets.

Since blood glucose is the essential or physiological sugar that is used as energy by our brains (as well as by parts of the eye and by muscle tissue during anaerobic conditions) and for many other biochemical reactions that take place in our bodies, it would seem that the more quickly this sugar could get into our blood, and from there to the tissues, the better off we would be. In fact, this is not the case, because normally we don't immediately need the large amount of energy provided by the intake of a sizable quantity of a simple sugar as, for example, in a candy bar. Our blood sugar (blood glucose) must be maintained in a fairly narrow range because if the level of glucose—which has other properties that can severely affect our physiology—is too high for too long, some serious problems can result, leading to death if not treated, as in the case of diabetes.

Insulin, a hormone produced by certain cells in the pancreas, regulates the levels of glucose in our blood. (Type I diabetics have no insulin, while type II diabetics—or adult onset—have an increased resistance to insulin, requiring a greater than normal amount to maintain their blood sugar in the required range.) Assuming we don't have diabetes, when we eat a candy bar or other source of simple sugar several sequential events occur. First, the simple sugars are quickly digested and are converted to blood glucose. Next, the blood glucose level is rapidly elevated, which stimulates the pancreas to release insulin. As the blood level of insulin increases, it causes the excess glucose to be moved from the blood into the cells where it is accumulated as glycogen (a storage form of glucose). Although the blood sugar level gradually returns to normal, the level of insulin remains elevated because insulin is metabolized more slowly. Persistently elevated insulin levels—usually incurred by chronic overconsumption of carbohydrates, type II diabetes, and obesity—cause several significant physiological repercussions including, but not limited to, the increased storage of fat and high blood pressure. In fact, let's look at how insulin affects the storage of fat and sugar.

First, let's discuss the way the body can use sugars that come from the diet, and the insulin response, if involved. These sugars can be:

1. used as a source of energy for the brain and other tissues. Insulin causes the body to lean toward the use of glucose for energy rather than fat. When insulin levels are low, the body tends to get most of its energy from the breakdown of fat—a situation we want to encourage.

2. stored as glycogen. As we have seen, increased levels of insulin cause the transfer of glucose into the cells where it is stored as glycogen. This glycogen can then be used directly as energy or converted back to glucose if necessary.

3. converted to other substances necessary to proper functioning of the body. Heparin, which prevents blood clotting, and many other vital biochemical entities are made from the glucose molecule.

4. converted to fat. Insulin increases the conversion of glucose to triglyceride and then to fat. Low levels of insulin make the system work in reverse, and fat is broken down and released to the tissues for energy—this is the desirable situation since it is fat we are trying to rid ourselves of.

5. converted to nonessential amino acids. The glucose molecule can be used in the liver to combine with protein-breakdown products to produce these nonessential amino acids.

As can be seen from the above, high levels of insulin favor the conversion of glucose to fat and tend to keep fat tissue from being broken down and used for energy. Low levels of insulin do the reverse. When insulin levels are down, the fat stores of the body are liberated and burned as fuel. It is easy to see that if we are trying to get rid of body fat, we should try to keep our insulin levels low so that our bodies get rid of this fat more efficiently. In my opinion, the best way to keep insulin levels low—a desirable situation—is with a carbohydrate-restricted diet.

Insulin also affects many other reactions in the body. It causes the kidneys to retain sodium, often leading to high blood pressure, and it increases the rate at which the body synthesizes cholesterol. We will discuss all these effects and their mechanisms in detail in a later chapter, but suffice it to say that the unrestrained consumption of carbohydrates—especially simple sugars—and the resulting chronic elevation of insulin is not without consequence.

Are Complex Carbohydrates Better?

Complex carbohydrates are either a mixture of starches and fiber, or as defined here, solely starches. Starches are nothing more than many simple sugars (often thousands) bound together in a manner that requires enzymatic breakdown by our digestive system to release these sugars. You can prove this to yourself by a simple experiment. Place in your mouth a small piece of a dry, white cracker, and chew it slowly. At first, the cracker will taste bland because it is primarily starch—for which we have no taste receptors, but as you continue to chew, it will start to taste sweeter and sweeter. Our saliva contains enzymes—the first of many to act upon food in our digestive tracts—that break down the starch into its component sugars, which, with our taste receptors for sweetness, we now perceive as sweet.

The primary difference between simple sugars and starches is that the starches take slightly longer to be broken down to reach their final product—blood glucose—and they generally don't produce the same magnitude of blood glucose levels as do simple sugars alone. This difference also results in an insulin response to starches that is typically more gradual, and usually not as pronounced. Diabetic patients do much better on diets that are high in starches instead of simple sugars because the slower release of glucose into their blood as the starches break down can be tolerated better by their insulin-deficient systems. The process is further complicated by the fact that different sugars and different starches—even when consumed on a gram-for-gram-equivalent-carbohydrate basis—produce markedly different increases in the blood glucose response.

Researchers have attempted to define this difference in glucose response by examining the rise in blood glucose produced by the consumption of various carbohydrate-containing foods. Subjects were first given 100 grams of glucose orally, then the degree of elevation of their blood glucose was measured over time—the standard "glucose tolerance test." The elevation of blood glucose generated by this oral glucose load was arbitrarily set at 100. Other carbohydrates are then evaluated in the same manner. Subjects consumed 100 grams of carbohydrate as corn, bread, sucrose, honey, ice cream, or any of a multitude of other items. The resulting elevation in blood glucose was then evaluated and compared to that caused by 100 grams of oral glucose alone. The comparison of the different responses is called the *glycemic index* and is calculated as follows: if

100 grams of sucrose (table sugar) produce a rise in the blood glucose that is equivalent to that produced by the 100 grams of glucose, the sucrose is said to have a glycemic index of 100; if, however, it produces a rise of only 50 percent of that caused by the glucose, then it has a glycemic index of 50. (Sucrose actually has a glycemic index of approximately 60.)

As far as diabetics are concerned, certain very low glycemic-index carbohydrates—certain legumes, for example—produce much less blood sugar elevation, and consequently less need for the administration of insulin. For the rest of us, since chronic elevations of our own insulin should be avoided, it makes sense to try to consume as many of our carbohydrates in a low-glycemic form as we can. In later chapters we will address this issue in more detail, and I will provide a different method of counting carbohydrates that leads to the selection of foods with a low glycemic index. Research in this area is far from complete, and since all glycemic indices are derived from results obtained by averaging the responses of many individuals, the figures may not hold true for all individuals to the same degree. At this point, investigators are trying to determine the effect that disparate glycemic-index foods have when eaten together. Do the glycemic indices average, and do fats and protein, when consumed together with carbohydrates, have a blunting effect? These are some of the questions currently being studied.

Fiber: The Indigestible Carbohydrate

A large portion of Chapter 10 will be devoted to an in-depth discussion of fiber, but now let's consider it briefly in order to compare it with the other forms of carbohydrate. Fiber comes in several forms—cellulose, hemicelluloses, pectin, lignins (the only noncarbohydrate fiber), gums, and mucilages—and is distinguished by the fact that humans do not have the capability of digesting it. Fiber can be divided into two main categories—soluble (can be dissolved in water) and insoluble (cannot be dissolved in water). All the recently described cholesterol- and blood-sugar-lowering effects attributed to fiber are properties of soluble fiber, while the property most people associate with fiber—stool bulking—is a function of insoluble fiber. The fiber found in oat bran, psyllium, fruits, and vegetables is mainly of the soluble variety, and bran and whole wheat contain insoluble fiber.

Cellulose, a common insoluble fiber found in bran and many other plant sources, is nothing more than several thousand glucose molecules hooked together, but in a way that humans cannot digest. It is basically the same structure as a starch, except that with starches we have digestive enzymes to break the bond holding the sugars together; we have no such enzymes to cleave the sugars in cellulose. Cows and other ruminants have the necessary enzyme and can derive energy from cellulose, but we can't. There are several companies that are currently producing pure cellulose—usually from wood—that is being used in bakery goods to replace a portion of the flour. This cellulose has many of the same baking properties of flour but has no calories or carbohydrates, and therefore, it reduces the total amount of these by 20 to 30 percent. Since, as we shall see, we get far too many carbohydrates in our typical diets, and far too little fiber, this substitution is beneficial since it replaces the former with the latter. I find it amusing to observe the various baking companies who are not using this cellulose decry those that are by saying they fill their bread products with "wood chips." Cellulose is cellulose whether it comes from wood or from wheat, just as vitamin C is the same whether acquired from orange juice or synthesized in a laboratory.

Fiber is sometimes listed on food labels and sometimes not. The breakfast cereal companies are doing an excellent job of labeling their products in terms of carbohydrates; the labels list the amount of simple sugars, complex sugars, and fiber. I wish that all food manufacturers would follow their lead. Often, fiber is listed on the label as carbohydrate, which is technically correct, but misleading. For example, the label on a specific food product may list its carbohydrate content as being 18 grams per serving, while in fact, of these 18 grams only 11 are simple and complex sugars, the remaining 7 grams being fiber. In accordance with new federal guidelines, the manufacturers must include fiber as a part of the total carbohydrate of the product, but they may list it separately as well. Under these regulations, a product containing 11 grams of fiber along with 20 grams of simple and complex sugars per serving could be labeled in two ways: it could read "31 grams of carbohydrate per serving" and nothing else, or it could be labeled "31 grams of carbohydrate, 11 grams fiber per serving." The regulating agencies confuse matters even more by permitting the food manufacturers to continue to label the old way—which allowed removal of the fiber amount from total carbohydrate—until their supply of printed labels is depleted. Manufacturers must abide by the new guidelines only when printing new labels. About the only way—until all labeling becomes uniform—to correctly tell the amount of fiber in any food is to purchase a book with the fiber contents of various foods listed. As an aside to all this, you should be aware of the distinction between "crude fiber" and "dietary fiber." "Crude fiber" is an out-of-date term that indicates the amount of fiber remaining after a food sample has artificially been digested by potent chemicals in the test laboratory. The newer tests more accurately approximate the human digestive system, and the amount of residue left over after these chemical digestions is referred to as "dietary fiber," a much more accurate term.

This may all seem like hairsplitting, but actually it is important in the diet you are about to embark upon. Since fiber is inert digestively, it doesn't figure into any carbohydrate counting plans. Only the actual simple and complex sugars that your body can use exert any carbohydrate effect—not the fiber. A food that contains 40 grams of carbohydrate, of which half is fiber, would contain only 20 grams of usable carbohydrate. If we are restricting ourselves to 50 grams of carbohydrate daily, we are interested in restricting only the true carbohydrate and not the fiber—especially not the fiber, because it, as we shall see, even exerts a blunting effect on the insulin-generating properties of sugar and starch.

Vitamins, Minerals, and Electrolytes

Now let's briefly examine the basic facts concerning vitamins and minerals in order to see how they fit into the various diet formats.

What is a vitamin? If asked this question, most people would be hard-pressed to come up with an answer. Vitamins, according to the average consumer, are capsules purchased in health food stores that, somehow, bring about an improvement in one's health after they are swallowed. In actuality, they are quite different. Vitamins are micronutrients (needed in very small amounts) that must be obtained from the diet, and they are organic chemicals (not minerals) that are available as a natural part of some foods. The consumption of vitamins does not necessarily generate good health, but deficiencies of vitamins can cause disease. In fact, vitamins were discovered as a result of the deficiency diseases—scurvy, pellagra,

beriberi, and others—that their absence brought about. People suffered these diseases even while consuming adequate amounts of
protein, carbohydrate, and fat; therefore, vitamins are not one of
these forms but are noncaloric chemicals. Vitamins, therefore, are
only necessary in very small amounts and should be obtained if at
all possible by eating foods rich in the required nutrients. Often, in
diets for weight reduction, certain foods are either severely restricted
or are eliminated altogether, and vitamin deficiencies can occur. In
these situations, which are of limited duration, vitamin supplements
should be taken. Also, I don't see any danger to people who take
a single balanced multivitamin supplement daily, even while not
on a weight reduction regimen, but I recommend against the consumption of large doses of single vitamins. There is an intricate
interplay between the various vitamins and minerals, with one,
consumed in overabundance, sometimes binding to another and
leading to a deficiency in the latter.

I don't mean to say that large dose or "mega" vitamin supplementation is not sometimes appropriate therapy for a specific disorder, but when given in such doses, it is administered as a drug
and not as a nutrient. Since "mega" doses of vitamins are drugs,
they should be given only under the supervision of a physician
skilled in their administration and aware of their potential for harm.
For our purposes, vitamins will be considered nutrients required in
very small amounts to maintain health, and not as "mega dose"
drugs.

There is absolutely no difference—either in chemical structure
or in physiological activity—between manufactured vitamins and
those found in food or other "natural" sources. Why then, if there
is no difference, does it matter whether we get our vitamins from
food or pills as long as we get them in adequate amounts? As far
as the vitamins are concerned, there is no difference. But a diet rich
in all the necessary vitamins and minerals will also be rich in all
the trace elements—chromium, selenium, molybdenum, and
others—the need for which may not yet have been established, and
rich in others perhaps that have not yet been identified.

A number of minerals—calcium, iron, iodine, magnesium, zinc,
and others—must be consumed in adequate amounts for the maintenance of health. Minerals differ from vitamins in that minerals are
elemental substances, usually used structurally, or to maintain electrical balance, whereas vitamins are complex chemically structured
substances used by the body mainly to facilitate biochemical reac-

tions. Minerals, in most cases, are required by the body in much larger quantities than are vitamins. For example, there are about three pounds of calcium in the body of an average-size person compared to only 0.05 to 0.1 ounces of vitamin C—a vitamin found in the human body in relatively large amounts. Both are necessary for good health; both should be obtained from food as much as possible.

Electrolytes are also elemental minerals, but they serve a different function from those mentioned above. The primary electrolytes in our bodies are sodium, potassium, and chloride, with sodium and chloride being the primary electrolytes in the fluids outside the cells, while potassium is found in high concentration mainly inside the cells. Electrolytes cannot be synthesized in the body and must come from dietary sources. The primary function of electrolytes is to maintain our bodies in electrical and osmotic (having to do with concentration gradients) equilibrium. In the absence of disorders such as chronic severe diarrhea, persistent vomiting, or diabetic acidosis, electrolyte deficiencies are unlikely. Deficiencies can be caused, however, by the use of diuretics in the absence of proper supplementation. It is possible to have an overabundance of electrolytes—most notably sodium—due to dietary excess. When the body has excess sodium, in order to maintain its concentration at normal levels, extra water must be retained. Sometimes this extra volume can cause high blood pressure, which may be treated with diuretics, which remove the excess sodium via the urine. Unfortunately, this treatment also removes potassium, which usually isn't present in excess and can cause deficiencies that, if not treated, can lead to fatigue, muscle weakness, and cramping, and in severe cases cardiac arrhythmia and even death. It is vitally important for you to either take potassium supplements or to make sure you have adequate dietary intake of potassium if you are undergoing a diuresis brought about by either medications or a dietary regimen such as the PSMF.

Calories

Calories are simply units of energy. Specifically, a calorie is the amount of heat (or energy) required to raise the temperature of one gram of water one degree Celsius. One thousand calories, or one kcal, equals one dietary calorie. Some books use a capital C for the dietary kind, Calorie, while others, mainly medical texts and journals, use kcal. Throughout this book, any mention of calories, capitalized or not, refers to the dietary variety. In a dietary context, calories are the amount of energy available in various foods. Protein and carbohydrate both contain 4 calories per gram (114 calories per ounce), fat contains 9 calories per gram (257 calories per ounce), and alcohol, 7 calories per gram (200 calories per ounce). The caloric content of a specific food tells us the amount of energy in that food that is *available* to us—not necessarily the amount of energy we will extract from it. The calories available are determined in test labs with the use of a calorimeter. The food in question is weighed and placed in the calorimeter where it is then heated in the presence of oxygen and completely burned to ash. By measuring the amount of oxygen required to accomplish this burning, the number of calories contained in the food can be determined. This number is modified by factors that have been obtained in laboratories from digestibility experiments, and the final result is the dietary calorie content of the food.

Calories are merely a measure of the amount of energy available, not the energy actually derived by the body from a specific food. The ability of the body to use the calories as energy is dependent upon the food's being absorbed from the intestinal tract. This absorption is dependent to a great extent on the particular food combinations eaten—often fiber interferes with the absorption of certain foods, making high-fiber diets less absorbable. Since fiber also is not digested, the caloric contribution of fiber is difficult to assess. What does this mean in terms of the energy content or weight-adding properties of our food? It means that, basically, a calorie is not always a calorie.

Obviously, a person consuming a 4,000-calorie-per-day diet composed of pork chops, mashed potatoes, and gravy would be more prone to gain weight than if he consumed a 2,000-calorie-per-day diet of the same composition but of one-half the portions. A 4,000-calorie-per-day diet made of pork chops alone, or of nothing but 4,000 calories worth of watermelon, may or may not cause an increased weight gain, since the number of usable calories is a function of both the type of food and the combinations of food consumed. If you increase or decrease the quantities of the same foods you always eat, you will either gain or lose weight (the more you add, the more weight you gain, and vice versa), but when you start changing the composition of the diet, all bets are off.

Let's use a low-carbohydrate diet—in this instance one that

contains 20 grams of carbohydrate per day—to demonstrate this effect. Even if this 20-gram diet contains 3,000 calories of energy, you will probably still lose weight, although not rapidly. If, on the other hand, this 20-gram diet contains only 1,000 calories of energy, you should lose much more rapidly. This is exactly what happens on the PSMF—it is a low-carbohydrate, low-calorie diet that maximizes the rate at which you lose body fat.

Dietary Guidelines

Several sets of criteria exist to help in the determination of the adequacy of any given dietary regimen. Two primary ones are in common usage—the Recommended Dietary Allowances (RDA), and the United States Recommended Daily Allowances (U.S. RDA). The RDAs set by the National Academy of Sciences are in their words "the levels of intake of essential nutrients considered in the judgment of the Committee on Dietary Allowances of the Food and Nutrition Board on the basis of available knowledge, to be adequate to meet the known nutritional needs of practically all healthy persons." These were last formulated in 1980 and are listed in Table 3.1. As you can see from this table, the RDAs provide information about all the nutrient requirements for males and females of several different age groups—fifteen categories in all plus extra categories for females who are pregnant or lactating.

The U.S. RDAs are nutrient standards set by the Food and Drug Administration (FDA) based upon the Recommended Dietary Allowances described above. The FDA has taken the RDA category with the highest requirement for each specific nutrient and made the nutrient requirement for that category the U.S. RDA. For example, males from the age of 19 to 22 is the RDA age/sex category requiring the most thiamine—1.5 mg per day; males from the age of 15 through 18 is the category requiring the most magnesium—400 mg per day. Thus, the U.S. RDA for thiamine is 1.5 mg per day, and for magnesium, 400 mg per day. There are no age or sex categories in the U.S. RDAs. Since for each nutrient category the maximum RDA amount is listed, if you consume that amount daily, you will be getting an adequate amount of that nutrient regardless of your age or sex. The U.S RDAs were set up in this fashion so that they could be used on food and vitamin labels—using the fifteen categories of the RDAs would be very cumbersome. On food labels,

TABLE 3.1

Food and Nutrition Board, National Academy of Sciences—National Research Council

Recommended Daily Dietary Allowances,[a] Revised 1980

Designed for the Maintenance of Good Nutrition of Practically All Healthy People in the U.S.A.

	Age (years)	Weight (kg)	Weight (lbs)	Height (cm)	Height (in)	Protein (g)	Fat-Soluble Vitamins			Water-Soluble Vitamins							Minerals					
							Vitamin A (µg)[b]	Vitamin D (µg)[c]	Vitamin E (mg α)[d]	Vitamin C (mg)	Thiamine (mg)	Riboflavin (mg)	Niacin (mg NE)[e]	Vitamin B6 (mg)	Folacin[f] (µg)	Vitamin B12 (µg)	Calcium (mg)	Phosphorus (mg)	Magnesium (mg)	Iron (mg)	Zinc (mg)	Iodine (µg)
Infants	0.0–0.5	6	13	60	24	kg × 2.2	420	10	3	35	0.3	0.4	6	0.3	30	0.5[g]	360	240	50	10	3	40
	0.5–1.0	9	20	71	28	kg × 2.0	400	10	4	35	0.5	0.6	8	0.6	45	1.5	540	360	70	15	5	50
Children	1–3	13	29	90	35	23	400	10	5	45	0.7	0.8	9	0.9	100	2.0	800	800	150	15	10	70
	4–6	20	44	112	44	30	500	10	6	45	0.9	1.0	11	1.3	200	2.5	800	800	200	10	10	90
	7–10	28	62	132	52	34	700	10	7	45	1.2	1.4	16	1.6	300	3.0	800	800	250	10	10	120
Males	11–14	45	99	157	62	45	1000	10	8	50	1.4	1.6	18	1.8	400	3.0	1200	1200	350	18	15	150
	15–18	66	145	176	69	56	1000	10	10	60	1.4	1.7	18	2.0	400	3.0	1200	1200	400	18	15	150
	19–22	70	154	177	70	56	1000	7.5	10	60	1.5	1.7	19	2.2	400	3.0	800	800	350	10	15	150
	23–50	70	154	178	70	56	1000	5	10	60	1.4	1.6	18	2.2	400	3.0	800	800	350	10	15	150
	51+	70	154	178	70	56	1000	5	10	60	1.2	1.4	16	2.2	400	3.0	800	800	350	10	15	150

Females	11–14	46	101	157	62	46	800	10	8	50	1.1	1.3	15	1.8	400	3.0	1200	1200	300	18	15	150
	15–18	55	120	163	64	46	800	10	8	60	1.1	1.3	14	2.0	400	3.0	1200	1200	300	18	15	150
	19–22	55	120	163	64	44	800	7.5	8	60	1.1	1.3	14	2.0	400	3.0	800	800	300	18	15	150
	23–50	55	120	163	64	44	800	5	8	60	1.0	1.2	13	2.0	400	3.0	800	800	300	18	15	150
	51+	55	120	163	64	44	800	5	8	60	1.0	1.2	13	2.0	400	3.0	800	800	300	10	15	150
Pregnant						+30	+200	+5	+2	+20	+0.4	+0.3	+2	+0.6	+400	+1.0	+400	+400	+150	[h]	+5	+25
Lactating						+20	+400	+5	+3	+40	+0.5	+0.5	+5	+0.5	+100	+1.0	+400	+400	+150	[h]	+10	+50

[a] The allowances are intended to provide for individual variations among most normal persons as they live in the United States under usual environmental stresses. Diets should be based on a variety of common foods in order to provide other nutrients for which human requirements have been less well defined.

[b] Retinol equivalents. 1 Retinol equivalent = 1 µg retinol or 6 µg β carotene.

[c] As cholecalciferol. 10 µg cholecalciferol = 400 IU vitamin D.

[d] α-tocopherol equivalents. 1 mg d-α-tocopherol = 1 α TE.

[e] 1 NE (niacin equivalent) is equal to 1 mg of niacin or 60 mg of dietary tryptophan.

[f] The folacin allowances refer to dietary sources as determined by *Lactobacillus casei* assay after treatment with enzymes (conjugases) to make polyglutamyl forms of the vitamin available to the test organism.

[g] The RDA for Vitamin B_{12} in infants is based on average concentration of the vitamin in human milk. The allowances after weaning are based on energy intake (as recommended by the American Academy of Pediatrics) and consideration of other factors such as intestinal absorption.

[h] The increased requirement during pregnancy cannot be met by the iron content of habitual American diets nor by the existing iron stores of many women; therefore the use of 30–60 mg of supplemental iron is recommended. Iron needs during lactation are not substantially different from those of nonpregnant women, but continued supplementation of the mother for 2–3 months after parturition is advisable in order to replenish stores depleted by pregnancy.

Reproduced from National Academy of Sciences: Recommended Dietary Allowances, 9th rev. ed. Washington, DC, 1980.

TABLE 3.2

United States Recommended Daily Allowances (U.S. RDA)[a]

	Unit	Infants (birth–12 mo.)	Children under 4 yrs.	Adults and children 4 or more yrs.	Pregnant or lactating women
Protein[b]	g	25	28	65	—
Protein[c]	g	18	20	45	—
Vitamin A	IU	1500	2500	5000	8000
Vitamin D	IU	400	400	400	400
Vitamin E	IU	5	10	30	30
Vitamin C	mg	35	40	60	60
Folic Acid	mg	0.1	0.2	0.4	0.8
Thiamine (B_1)	mg	0.5	0.7	1.5	1.7
Riboflavin (B_2)	mg	0.6	0.8	1.7	2.0
Niacin	mg	8	9	20	20
Vitamin B_6	mg	0.4	0.7	2.0	2.5
Vitamin B_{12}	mcg	2	3	6	8
Biotin	mg	0.05	0.15	0.3	0.3
Pantothenic Acid	mg	3	5	10	10
Calcium	g	0.6	0.8	1.0	1.3
Phosphorus	g	0.5	0.8	1.0	1.3
Iodine	mcg	45	70	150	150
Iron	mg	15	10	18	18
Magnesium	mg	70	200	400	450
Copper	mg	0.6	1.0	2.0	2.0
Zinc	mg	5	8	15	15

[a] The U.S. RDAs are nutrient standards set by the Food and Drug Administration in 1973 using the Recommended Dietary Allowances of the National Academy of Sciences, National Research Council. The U.S. RDAs are established for four age–sex groups. Generally, the highest values in the RDA table were selected for use within each U.S. RDA category. The nutritional information on food labels is expressed as percent of the U.S. RDA.

[b] Protein efficiency ratio less than casein.

[c] Protein efficiency ratio greater than or equal to casein.

Reproduced from the FDA consumer memo, "Nutrition Labels and U.S. RDA." 81-2146, 1981.

the nutritional information is expressed as a percentage of the U.S. RDA. The U.S. RDAs are listed in Table 3.2.

Types of Diets

Now that we have discussed the various types of food substances and the dietary guidelines, let's look at how the commonly used dietary regimens for weight loss fit these criteria. Let us examine first the typical American diet, then see how it is modified to become a weight-loss diet. Assuming that the average American—not on a diet—consumes around 2,500 calories per day, how are these calories allocated among the food groups? Table 3.3 shows this allocation in tabular form.

Low-Calorie Diets

Low-calorie diets are without a doubt the most commonly used for weight loss. In these diets, the number of calories (or available energy) is restricted so that the dieter will have to use his body reserves (fat) to provide the necessary energy needed to maintain life. There is no doubt that restricting the caloric intake to low levels will promote weight loss, but is it a healthy weight loss? In typical low-calorie diets composed primarily of fruits and vegetables, the caloric restriction comes mainly from the reduction of fat. If we reduce our total calories from 2,500 per day to 1,500, giving a 1,000-calorie daily deficit, we should lose weight. (If we reduce our fat intake to 20 percent of these calories, we will be consuming 300

T A B L E 3.3

Food Group Allocation of the Typical
2,500-Calorie American Diet

Protein	12%	300 Cal	75 grams
Carbohydrate	45%	1125 Cal	280 grams*
Fat	42%	1050 Cal	116 grams

*includes approximately 125 grams of refined sugar

TABLE 3.4

Composition of 1,500-Calorie Weight-Reduction Diet

Protein	13%	200 Cal	50 grams
Carbohydrate	67%	1000 Cal	250 grams
Fat	20%	300 Cal	33 grams

calories—33 grams—as fat. Some low-calorie diets restrict fat even further—to 15 or even 10 percent of calories—but these diets are not very palatable and most people cannot tolerate them for long periods. Let's construct our various diets in a way that is palatable and satisfying on a long-term basis.) Unfortunately, the reduction of fat is usually accompanied by a reduction in protein, since they are often found in foods together. While we are reducing our intake of fat by greater than 70 percent, from 116 grams to 33 grams, if we only reduce our protein by one-third, we are left with 50 grams of protein—by the U.S. RDA, an inadequate amount for adults, causing a deficiency of 15 grams of protein per day.

This potential for protein inadequacy points out a problem with low-calorie diets—often muscle mass is lost. Muscle is lost on a low-calorie diet in approximately the same proportion as it is on a complete fast—just not as quickly. Typically, 30 to 40 percent of the weight lost on low-calorie diets is from lean-body weight.

Of the 1,000-calorie deficit we are seeking, 750 calories come from the reduction of fat intake and another 100 calories from lowered protein, leaving 150 calories that must be removed as carbohydrates. By reducing the intake of refined sugar by 38 grams or approximately 30 percent, this can be done. The composition of our low-calorie diet appears in Table 3.4.

Low-Carbohydrate Diets

On low-carbohydrate diets, only carbohydrate is restricted. If we eliminate all carbohydrates—which are nutritionally nonessential—from our diets, we can rid ourselves of 1,125 calories, while continuing to eat everything else in the typical American diet. Although limited in variety, a diet without carbohydrate would be infinitely more palatable than a diet without fat. But we don't have to eliminate all carbohydrates. If we just eliminate all refined sugar, we reduce our calories by 500. If we restrict our total carbohydrate intake to 60 grams per day—enough to provide a variety of fruits and vegetables—we remove 885 calories from our diet.

Surprisingly, by restricting carbohydrate intake, we also restrict our intake of fat because many foods that we are used to thinking of only in terms of sugar content are loaded with fat as well. Candy bars, ice cream, pastries, french fries, malts—all are loaded with fat along with carbohydrate. If we eliminate these foods, and others like them, from our diet in order to decrease our carbohydrate consumption, we will eliminate considerable fat at the same time. The most mistaken notion about a low-carbohydrate diet is that it is also a high-fat diet. Granted, it is not as low in fat as a typical low-calorie diet, but it is lower in fat than the typical American diet.

If in addition to reducing our carbohydrate intake to 60 grams per day, we increase our protein intake to 100 grams, we can account for only 640 calories from these foods. To get our 1,500 calories, we must consume 96 grams or 860 calories of fat—a decrease of 20 grams from the typical diet. The composition of the low-carbohydrate diet is listed in Table 3.5.

These figures have been manipulated a little to make the total calories come out to 1,500. In actuality, the total calories would probably be fewer than that, but for comparison I set both diets at 1,500 calories. The nice thing about being on a low-carbohydrate diet is that you don't really have the feeling that you are dieting. Whenever you are given unlimited access to almost any food components, it removes the onus of dieting, since dieting, by definition, is the restriction of food.

Low-carbohydrate diets are more than adequate in protein while low-calorie diets are often inadequate. Extremely low-calorie/low-fat diets such as the Pritikin can bring about deficiencies in essential fatty acids. As we will see in Chapter 8, the low-carbohydrate diet

T A B L E 3.5

Composition of a 1,500-Calorie Low-Carbohydrate Diet

Protein	27%	400 Cal	100 grams
Carbohydrate	16%	240 Cal	60 grams
Fat	57%	860 Cal	96 grams

TABLE 3.6

Composition of 1,000-Calorie PSMF Diet

Protein	40%	400 Cal	100 grams
Carbohydrate	16%	160 Cal	40 grams
Fat	48%	480 Cal	53 grams

produces no similar deficiencies, and in fact more than exceeds the U.S. RDA in all categories.

Protein-Sparing Modified Fast

The PSMF is a diet that is strictly for weight loss, and it is lower in calories than the other two we have discussed. The protein supplements can be made in several forms—shakes, puddings, soups —and have varying amounts of the different nutrients. Because the supplements are generally made of a pure protein with a small amount of carbohydrate and fat added, it becomes necessary to have patients on the PSMF take vitamins and minerals in supplement form. This is not true with supplements manufactured commercially and provided by your physician, as these have all the necessary nutrients included; however, if you prepare your own, you must take vitamin supplements.

The PSMF protocol outlined in this book provides about 1,000 calories. Of these approximately 1,000 calories, 400 are from protein, 160 from carbohydrate, and 480 are from fat. The PSMF composition is listed in Table 3.6.

If you are on either the low-carbohydrate diet or the PSMF, you will maintain the majority of your lean-body weight and lose mainly fat. While it is possible to lose large amounts of weight on a low-carbohydrate diet, this feat is accomplished much more quickly on the PSMF. This is because the PSMF, while a low-carbohydrate/ high-protein diet, contains very few calories, whereas a low-carbohydrate diet (such as the maintenance diet I describe in Chapter 8) contains more calories. In the following chapter you will learn how to determine your lean-body weight, amount of body fat, and a method to derive your realistic goal weight.

4

Why Weight?

B^Y now, if you've studied the last chapter, you are brimming with nutritional knowledge. You know about complete proteins, you know that all fats aren't bad, and you know what a carbohydrate is and how the carbohydrate/insulin system works. You've learned what a vitamin is and why you don't need them in "mega" doses, and you now have a standard by which you can determine the nutritional adequacy of any dietary regimen—the RDA or the U.S. RDA. And lastly, you saw how the PSMF and the low-carbohydrate maintenance diet compare with the typical American diet, and with a standard low-calorie diet in terms of both protein adequacy and the amount of fat consumed. Many of your concerns about the health consequences of the PSMF should have been allayed in Chapter 3—the rest will be addressed in Chapters 10 and 11. I know you're ready to blast off into the actual diet, so let's go. The first thing you need to do is to get your starting weight. Or is it?

When you start this or any other diet program, you need some means of monitoring your progress. You need to know what your starting point is, what your goal is, and a plan for checking yourself along the way. Most people do this by tracking their weight—a simple procedure. But unfortunately, not a very precise method, and one that often leads to much disappointment. In this chapter, you will learn a much more accurate way to judge your starting point, goal, and progress—by measuring the actual amount of excess fat you are "wearing." Let's look first at what you've probably done in the past, what most dieters continue to do, and why it doesn't really make sense.

When in the past you've decided to embark upon a diet, the first step you probably took was to jump on the scales to obtain your starting weight. As the diet continued, you monitored your progress by the fluctuation of your weight as measured by the scales. You may have had special schedules worked out whereby you only weighed on certain days, or you may have weighed daily, but whatever scheme you used, you—as all dieters do—rated the success or failure of your diet by the amount of weight you lost—or didn't lose—as measured by the scales. Delight, frustration, rage, ecstasy, and disappointment are just a few of the emotions you may have experienced due to the reading on the bathroom scales. This weighing compulsion would be appropriate except for the fact that you really didn't diet to lose weight; you dieted to lose excess fat. And since our society so focuses upon weight as the key, throughout this book when I refer to losing *weight*, I really mean losing *fat*.

We are all attuned to our weight because it is so easily measured, but these bathroom-scale readings can be very deceiving. The scales measure weight but do not tell if the weight is due to a large bone structure, heavy muscularity, excess fluid retention, or a combination of these factors. In other words, the scales don't measure size, but size is what we are concerned with. We all talk about how much weight we lost on a particular diet, but what we really mean is how much size we lost. I always tell my patients that it doesn't matter if they weigh 280 pounds as long as they can fit into a size 6. I am being facetious, of course, since no one who weighs 280 pounds could possibly wear a size 6, but the principle is valid. People should be much more concerned about their size than about their weight; our size is what constitutes our appearance, whether it be overweight or underweight. If someone looks at us, they don't see our weight, but they do see our size. Excess size is a result of excess fat. Excess fat is what makes us not only appear unhealthy but actually be unhealthy. Since the health problems and the aesthetic problems all arise from the excess fat, doesn't it seem reasonable that we should attempt to measure body fat as an index of obesity rather than measure weight?

Who would consider Arnold Schwarzenegger obese? The Metropolitan Life Insurance Company would. According to their height/weight tables published in 1983, Mr. Schwarzenegger is 32 percent above his ideal body weight, and consequently, he is in jeopardy of serious health problems. Accordingly, by their standards, he is at high risk for diabetes, heart disease, and multiple forms of cancer, and if he were wise, he would take immediate steps to reduce this excess weight. This is all nonsense of course as Mr. Schwarzenegger is an exceptionally well-developed, very muscular, highly trained athlete who is undoubtedly in exceedingly good health. His case illustrates, however, that we cannot determine who is or isn't excessively fat based upon weight alone.

The proper method to determine the degree to which you are overweight is by measuring the amount of body fat you have in excess of what you should have. This is done by determining the percentage of your weight that is fat—your body fat percentage. Just as there are tables listing the "desirable" weights for varying heights and frame sizes, there are tables listing the optimal body fat percentages as a function of age and sex. One such table is Table 4.1.

From this table you can see that a female, age 33, should carry from 21 to 27 percent body fat irrespective of her height or frame size. What does this tell us and how does this help us lose size? We can find what our ideal body fat percentage *should be* from Table 4.1, but in order to make this table a useful tool, we must be able to determine what our percentage is now. Only then can we know how much fat we need to lose.

TABLE 4.1

Optimal Body Fat Percentages

Age	Males	Females
10–30	12–18%	20–26%
31–40	13–19%	21–27%
41–50	14–20%	22–28%
51–60	16–20%	22–30%
61 and older	17–21%	22–31%

To determine how much of our weight is fat and how much lean, physicians use one of several techniques. Please refer to the simple schematic diagram below.

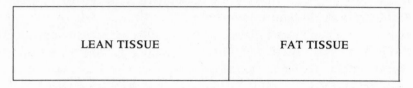

This diagram shows that our bodies are composed of basically two substances: fatty tissue and everything else, which we refer to collectively as lean body tissue. This lean body tissue is bone, muscle, nerve tissue, organs, and essentially anything that is not specifically fat. If, for instance, fat makes up 35 percent of our body weight, to determine lean body weight, we would simply need to subtract this 35 percent from 100 percent. The resultant figure—in this case 65 percent—would be the percent of our weight contributed by our lean or nonfat tissue. Either of these figures—the percent body fat or percent lean-body weight—can be multiplied times the patient's weight, and a number in pounds of fat or lean-body weight results. Then, by knowing the lean-body weight and adding to it the ideal percentage of fat from table 4.1, we can determine a realistic ideal body weight.

Measuring Body Fat

There are several methods of body composition measurement in use today. As with most procedures, increased accuracy and reliability comes with increased expense—some of the most accurate methods are suitable only for laboratory use. There are four types of measurement techniques in use currently: total body water measurement methods, hydrostatic weighing methods, bioelectrical impedance methods, and anthropometric methods.

Research laboratories often use the *total body water* measurement methods because of their accuracy, but the various procedures require much time and painstaking attention to detail. In these tests, the patient ingests some sort of chemically or radioactively "labeled" water. After several hours, the labeled water will have been absorbed, be evenly distributed in the body fluid space, and available for measurement by various devices. With these results, researchers are able to first calculate the total body water and its distribution, then with this knowledge determine the amounts of fat and lean tissue present.

Hydrostatic measurement has been the most widely used method of determining body composition. The person is first weighed standing on scales and then totally submersed in water and re-weighed in the water tank. By knowing the different densities of various body substances, researchers can determine the amounts of fat and lean body tissue. Hydrostatic measurements, while fairly accurate, are expensive and cause considerable inconvenience to the subject.

In my practice, I use the *bioelectrical impedance* method to mea-sure body composition. The nurse weighs the patient and measures his height. He then lies down and she attaches an electrode patch to his hand and foot. One of the electrodes, which is connected to a small computer, transmits a small electrical charge through the body to another electrode. The computer then measures the imped-ance of the patient's body, calculating the percentages of the various body tissues. Multiple studies have demonstrated a close correlation between bioelectrical impedance values and the values acquired by hydrostatic weighing. Except for the initial purchase of the necessary equipment, this technique is inexpensive to perform, takes just a few moments, and causes no discomfort to the patient.

Before I obtained the equipment for the bioelectrical impedance testing, I used anthropometric methods to determine the body composition of my patients. *Anthropometry* is the measurement of the body surface or thickness of skin at various points, and the correlation of these measurements with fat tissue mass and lean tissue weight. The equipment necessary—a tape measure or skin calipers—is inexpensive, and the actual measuring takes little time. Theoretically, this is the least accurate of the methods available, but when I started using the bioelectrical impedance procedure, I con-tinued to use the anthropometric technique concurrently to compare the two and found the differences to be insignificant. The results never varied by more than 2 percent and were often the same.

Determining Realistic Ideal Weight

In order to calculate your realistic ideal weight, you must know your percentage body fat. You can consult a physician or research center that does this type of measurement using one of the methods we discussed above, or you can do your own anthropometric determination using the tables in this book.

To use this technique—the same one I used in my practice for several years—you will need a tape measure, a scale, and Table 4.2 if you are female or Table 4.3 if you are male. You should make all measurements on bare skin (not through clothing), and make sure that the tape fits snugly but does not compress the skin and underlying tissue. Take all measurements three times and calculate the average. All measurements should be in inches.

Calculating Body Fat Percentages for Females

There are five steps you must take to calculate your percentage body fat:

1. While keeping the tape level, measure your hips at their widest point, and your waist at the umbilicus (belly button). It is critical that you measure at the umbilicus and *not* at the narrowest point of your waist. Take each of these measurements three times and compute an average for each.

2. Measure your height in inches without shoes.

3. Record your height, waist, and hip measurements in the labeled spaces on the worksheet on page 63.

4. Find each of these measurements in the appropriate column in Table 4.2 and record the adjacent constant on the worksheet. These constants have been derived experimentally and allow you to convert your measurements into a form that can be used to compute your percentage body fat.

5. Add constants A and B, then subtract constant C from this sum and round to the nearest whole number. This figure is your percentage body fat.

WORKSHEET—WOMEN
COMPUTING YOUR PERCENT BODY FAT

First, find your average measurements IN INCHES of:

	Hips	Abdomen	Height
measurement #1	___	___	___
+			
measurement #2	___	___	
+			
measurement #3	___	___	
total =	___	___	
divide by 3 =	___	___	___
	Constant A	Constant B	Consant C

Using Table 4.2, look up each of these average measurements and your height in the appropriate column. The numbers listed beside them will be Constant A (hips), Constant B (abdomen), and Constant C (height). Use these constants below:

Add together	_____	Constant A (hips)
+	_____	Constant B (abdomen)
	_____	
subtract −	_____	Constant C (height)
	_____	= your percent body fat

TABLE 4.2

Conversion Constants to Predict Percent Body Fat—Women

HIPS		ABDOMEN		HEIGHT	
Inches	Constant A	Inches	Constant B	Inches	Constant C
30	33.48	20	14.22	55	33.52
30.5	33.83	20.5	14.40	55.5	33.67
31	34.87	21	14.93	56	34.13
31.5	35.22	21.5	15.11	56.5	34.28
32	36.27	22	15.64	57	34.74
32.5	36.62	22.5	15.82	57.5	34.89
33	37.67	23	16.35	58	35.35
33.5	38.02	23.5	16.53	58.5	35.50
34	39.06	24	17.06	59	35.96
34.5	39.41	24.5	17.24	59.5	36.11
35	40.46	25	17.78	60	36.57
35.5	40.81	25.5	17.96	60.5	36.72
36	41.86	26	18.49	61	37.18
36.5	42.21	26.5	18.67	61.5	37.33
37	43.25	27	19.20	62	37.79
37.5	43.60	27.5	19.38	62.5	37.94
38	44.65	28	19.91	63	38.40
38.5	45.00	28.5	20.09	63.5	38.55

64	39.01	29	20.62	39	46.05
64.5	39.16	29.5	20.80	39.5	46.40
65	39.62	30	21.33	40	47.44
65.5	39.77	30.5	21.51	40.5	47.79
66	40.23	31	22.04	41	48.84
66.5	40.38	31.5	22.22	41.5	49.19
67	40.84	32	22.75	42	50.24
67.5	40.99	32.5	22.93	42.5	50.59
68	41.45	33	23.46	43	51.64
68.5	41.60	33.5	23.64	43.5	51.99
69	42.06	34	24.18	44	53.03
69.5	42.21	34.5	24.36	44.5	53.41
70	42.67	35	24.89	45	54.53
70.5	42.82	35.5	25.07	45.5	54.86
71	43.28	36	25.60	46	55.83
71.5	43.43	36.5	25.78	46.5	56.18
72	43.89	37	26.31	47	57.22
72.5	44.04	37.5	26.49	47.5	57.57
73	44.50	38	27.02	48	58.62
73.5	44.65	38.5	27.20	48.5	58.97
74	45.11	39	27.73	49	60.02
74.5	45.26	39.5	27.91	49.5	60.37
75	45.72	40	28.44	50	61.42
75.5	45.87	40.5	28.62	50.5	61.77
76	46.32	41	29.15	51	62.81

TABLE 4.2

Conversion Constants to Predict Percent Body Fat—Women

HIPS		ABDOMEN		HEIGHT	
Inches	Constant A	Inches	Constant B	Inches	Constant C
51.5	63.16	41.5	29.33	76.5	46.47
52	64.21	42	29.87	77	46.93
52.5	64.56	42.5	30.05	77.5	47.08
53	65.61	43	30.58	78	47.54
53.5	65.96	43.5	30.76	78.5	47.69
54	67.00	44	31.29	79	48.15
54.5	67.35	44.5	31.47	79.5	48.30
55	68.40	45	32.00	80	48.76
55.5	68.75	45.5	32.18	80.5	48.91
56	69.80	46	32.71	81	49.37
56.5	70.15	46.5	32.89	81.5	49.52
57	71.19	47	33.42	82	49.98
57.5	71.54	47.5	33.60	82.5	50.13
58	72.59	48	34.13	83	50.59
58.5	72.94	48.5	34.31	83.5	50.74
59	73.99	49	34.84	84	51.20
59.5	74.34	49.5	35.02	84.5	51.35
60	75.39	50	35.56	85	51.81

Calculating Body Fat Percentages for Men

There are four steps you must take to determine your body fat percentage:

1. While keeping the tape level, measure the circumference of your waist at the umbilicus (belly button). Measure three times and compute the average.

2. Measure your wrist at the space between your hand and your wrist bone, where your wrist bends.

3. Record these measurements on the worksheet for males on page 74.

4. Subtract your wrist measurement from your waist measurement and find the resultant value listed across the top of Table 4.3. On the left-hand side of this table, find your weight. Proceed to the right from your weight and down from your waist-minus-wrist measurement. Where these two points intersect, read your body fat percentage directly from the table beginning on page 68.

Calculating Lean-Body Weight

Now that you know your body fat percentage, the next step is to use this figure to compute your realistic ideal weight. The first step is to calculate the weight in pounds of the fat portion of your body. This is done by multiplying your weight by your percent body fat.

$$\text{weight} \times \text{\% body fat} = \text{weight of fat}$$

Once you know the weight of your body fat, you subtract that weight from your total weight to find your lean-body weight. Lean-body weight is the total weight of all nonfat body tissue.

$$\text{total weight} - \text{body fat weight} = \text{lean-body weight}$$

Now you have all the necessary numbers to determine your ideal body weight. Refer now to Table 4.1 to find the body fat percentage range that is appropriate for your age. Take the numbers

T A B L E 4.3

Waist-Minus-Wrist
Body Fat Calculation—Male

Waist Minus Wrist (in inches)

Weight in lbs.	22	22.5	23	23.5	24	24.5	25	25.5	26	26.5	27	27.5	28	28.5	29	29.5	30	30.5	31
120	4	6	8	10	12	14	16	18	20	21	23	25	27	29	31	33	35	37	39
125	4	6	7	9	11	13	15	17	19	20	22	24	26	28	30	32	33	35	37
130	3	5	7	9	11	12	14	16	18	20	21	23	25	27	28	30	32	34	36
135	3	5	7	8	10	12	13	15	17	19	20	22	24	26	27	29	31	32	34
140	3	5	6	8	10	11	13	15	16	18	19	21	23	24	26	28	29	31	33
145	3	4	6	7	9	11	12	14	15	17	19	20	22	23	25	27	28	30	31
150	2	4	6	7	9	10	12	13	15	16	18	19	21	23	24	26	27	29	30
155	2	4	5	6	8	10	11	13	14	16	17	19	20	22	23	25	26	28	29
160	2	4	5	6	8	9	11	12	14	15	17	18	19	21	22	24	25	27	28
165	2	3	5	6	8	9	10	12	13	15	16	17	19	20	22	23	24	26	27
170	2	3	4	6	7	9	10	11	13	14	15	17	18	19	21	22	24	25	26
175	2	3	4	6	7	8	10	11	12	13	15	16	17	19	20	21	23	24	25
180	1	3	4	5	7	8	9	10	12	13	14	16	17	18	19	21	22	23	25
185	1	3	4	5	6	8	9	10	11	13	14	15	16	18	19	20	21	23	24
190	1	2	4	5	6	7	8	10	11	12	13	15	16	17	18	19	21	22	23

Waist Minus Wrist (in inches)

Weight in lbs.	22	22.5	23	23.5	24	24.5	25	25.5	26	26.5	27	27.5	28	28.5	29	29.5	30	30.5	31
195	1	2	3	5	6	7	8	9	11	12	13	14	15	16	18	19	20	21	22
200	1	2	3	4	6	7	8	9	10	11	12	14	15	16	17	18	19	21	22
205	1	2	3	4	5	6	8	9	10	11	12	13	14	15	17	18	19	20	21
210	1	2	3	4	5	6	7	8	9	11	12	13	14	15	16	17	18	19	21
215	1	2	3	4	5	6	7	8	9	10	11	12	13	15	16	17	18	19	20
220	0	2	3	4	5	6	7	8	9	10	11	12	13	14	15	16	17	18	19
225	0	1	2	3	4	6	7	8	9	10	11	12	13	14	15	16	17	18	19
230	0	1	2	3	4	5	6	7	8	9	10	11	12	13	14	15	16	17	18
235	0	1	2	3	4	5	6	7	8	9	10	11	12	13	14	15	16	17	18
240	0	1	2	3	4	5	6	7	8	9	10	11	12	13	14	15	16	17	17
245	0	1	2	3	4	5	6	7	8	9	9	10	11	12	13	14	15	16	17
250	0	1	2	3	4	5	6	6	7	8	9	10	11	12	13	14	15	16	17
255	0	1	2	3	3	4	5	6	7	8	9	10	11	12	13	14	14	15	16
260	0	1	2	2	3	4	5	6	7	8	9	10	10	11	12	13	14	15	16
265	0	1	2	2	3	4	5	6	7	8	8	9	10	11	12	13	14	15	15
270	0	1	2	2	3	4	5	6	7	7	8	9	10	11	12	13	13	14	15
275	0	1	2	2	3	4	5	5	6	7	8	9	10	11	11	12	13	14	15
280	0	0	1	2	3	4	4	5	6	7	8	9	9	10	11	12	13	14	14
285	0	0	1	2	3	4	4	5	6	7	8	8	9	10	11	12	12	13	14
290	0	0	1	2	3	4	4	5	6	7	7	8	9	10	11	11	12	13	14
295	0	0	1	2	2	3	4	5	6	6	7	8	9	10	11	11	12	13	14
300	0	0	1	2	2	3	4	5	5	6	7	8	9	9	10	11	12	12	13

TABLE 4.3

Waist-Minus-Wrist
Body Fat Calculation—Male

Weight in lbs. \ Waist Minus Wrist (in inches)	31.5	32	32.5	33	33.5	34	34.5	35	35.5	36	36.5	37	37.5	38	38.5	39	39.5	40	40.5
120	41	43	45	47	49	50	52	54	56	58	60	62	64	66	68	70	70	74	76
125	39	41	43	45	46	48	50	52	54	56	58	59	61	63	65	67	69	71	72
130	37	39	41	43	44	46	48	50	52	53	55	57	59	61	62	64	66	68	69
135	36	38	39	41	43	44	46	48	50	51	53	55	56	58	60	62	63	68	67
140	34	36	38	39	41	43	44	46	48	49	51	53	54	56	58	59	61	63	64
145	33	35	36	38	39	41	43	44	46	47	49	51	52	54	55	57	59	60	62
150	32	33	35	36	38	40	41	43	44	46	47	49	50	52	53	55	57	58	60
155	31	32	34	35	37	38	40	41	43	44	46	47	49	50	52	53	55	56	58
160	30	31	33	34	35	37	38	40	41	43	44	46	47	48	50	51	53	54	56
165	29	30	31	33	34	36	37	38	40	41	43	44	45	47	48	50	51	52	54
170	28	29	30	32	33	34	36	37	39	40	41	43	44	45	47	48	49	51	52
175	27	28	29	31	32	33	35	36	37	39	40	41	43	44	45	47	48	49	51
180	26	27	28	30	31	32	34	35	36	37	39	40	41	43	44	45	47	48	49
185	25	26	28	29	30	31	33	34	35	36	38	39	40	41	43	44	45	46	48
190	24	26	27	28	29	30	32	33	34	35	37	38	39	40	41	43	44	45	46
195	24	25	26	27	28	30	31	32	33	34	35	37	38	39	40	41	43	44	45

Waist Minus Wrist
(in inches)

Weight in lbs.	31.5	32	32.5	33	33.5	34	34.5	35	35.5	36	36.5	37	37.5	38	38.5	39	39.5	40	40.5
200	23	24	25	26	28	29	30	31	32	33	35	36	37	38	39	40	41	43	44
205	22	23	25	26	27	28	29	30	31	32	34	35	36	37	38	39	40	41	43
210	22	23	24	25	26	27	28	29	30	32	33	34	35	36	37	38	39	40	42
215	21	22	23	24	25	26	28	29	30	31	32	33	34	35	36	37	38	39	40
220	20	22	23	24	25	26	27	28	29	30	31	32	33	34	35	36	37	38	39
225	20	21	22	23	24	25	26	27	28	29	30	31	32	33	34	35	36	37	38
230	19	20	21	22	23	24	25	26	27	28	30	31	32	33	34	35	36	37	38
235	19	20	21	22	23	24	25	26	27	28	29	30	31	32	33	34	35	36	37
240	18	19	20	21	22	23	24	25	26	27	28	29	30	31	32	33	34	35	36
245	18	19	20	21	22	23	24	25	26	27	27	28	29	30	31	32	33	34	35
250	18	18	19	20	21	22	23	24	25	26	27	28	29	30	31	31	32	33	34
255	17	18	19	20	21	22	23	24	24	25	26	27	28	29	30	31	32	33	34
260	17	18	19	19	20	21	22	23	24	25	26	27	27	28	29	30	31	32	33
265	16	17	18	19	20	21	22	22	23	24	25	26	27	28	29	29	30	31	32
270	16	17	18	19	19	20	21	22	23	24	25	25	26	27	28	29	30	31	31
275	16	16	17	18	19	20	21	22	22	23	24	25	26	27	27	28	29	30	31
280	15	16	17	18	19	19	20	21	22	23	24	24	25	26	27	28	29	30	30
285	15	16	17	17	18	19	20	21	21	22	23	24	25	26	26	27	28	29	30
290	15	15	16	17	18	19	19	20	21	22	23	23	24	25	26	27	27	29	29
295	14	15	16	17	17	18	19	20	21	21	22	23	24	25	25	26	27	28	28
300	14	15	16	16	17	18	19	19	20	21	22	22	23	24	25	26	26	28	28

TABLE 4.3

Waist-Minus-Wrist
Body Fat Calculation—Male

Weight in lbs.	Waist Minus Wrist (in inches): 41	41.5	42	42.5	43	43.5	44	44.5	45	45.5	46	46.5	47	47.5	48	48.5	49	49.5	50
120	77	79	81	83	85	87	89	91	93	95	97	99	99	99	99	99	99	99	99
125	74	76	78	80	82	84	85	87	89	91	93	95	96	98	99	99	99	99	99
130	71	73	75	77	78	80	82	84	86	87	89	91	93	94	96	98	99	99	99
135	68	70	72	74	75	77	79	80	82	84	86	87	89	91	92	94	96	98	99
140	66	68	69	71	72	74	76	77	79	81	82	84	86	87	89	91	92	94	96
145	63	65	67	68	70	71	73	75	76	78	79	81	83	84	86	87	89	91	92
150	61	63	64	66	67	69	70	72	74	75	77	78	80	81	83	84	86	87	89
155	59	61	62	64	65	67	68	70	71	73	74	76	77	79	80	82	83	85	86
160	57	59	60	61	63	64	66	67	69	70	72	73	75	76	77	79	80	82	83
165	55	57	58	60	61	62	64	65	67	68	69	71	72	74	75	76	78	79	81
170	54	55	56	58	59	60	62	63	64	66	67	69	70	71	73	74	75	77	78
175	52	53	55	56	57	59	60	61	63	64	65	66	68	69	70	72	73	74	76
180	50	52	53	54	56	57	58	59	61	62	63	65	66	67	68	70	71	72	74
185	49	50	51	53	54	55	56	58	59	60	61	63	64	65	66	68	69	70	71
190	48	49	50	51	52	54	55	56	57	58	60	61	62	63	65	66	67	68	69
195	46	47	49	50	51	52	53	55	56	57	58	59	60	62	63	64	65	66	68

Waist Minus Wrist
(in inches)

Weight in lbs.	41	41.5	42	42.5	43	43.5	44	44.5	45	45.5	46	46.5	47	47.5	48	48.5	49	49.5	50
200	45	46	47	48	50	51	52	53	54	55	57	58	59	60	61	62	63	65	66
205	44	45	46	47	48	49	51	52	53	54	55	56	57	58	60	61	62	63	64
210	43	44	45	46	47	48	49	50	51	53	54	55	56	57	58	59	60	61	62
215	42	43	44	45	46	47	48	49	50	51	52	53	54	56	57	58	59	60	61
220	41	42	43	44	45	46	47	48	49	50	51	52	53	54	55	56	57	58	59
225	40	41	42	43	44	45	46	47	48	49	50	51	52	53	54	55	56	57	58
230	39	40	41	42	43	44	45	46	47	48	49	50	51	52	53	54	55	56	57
235	38	39	40	41	42	43	44	45	46	47	48	49	50	51	51	52	53	54	55
240	37	38	39	40	41	42	43	44	45	46	46	47	48	49	50	51	52	53	54
245	36	37	38	39	40	41	42	43	44	44	45	46	47	48	49	50	51	52	53
250	35	36	37	38	39	40	41	42	43	44	44	45	46	47	48	49	50	51	52
255	34	35	36	37	38	39	40	41	42	43	44	44	45	46	47	48	49	50	51
260	34	35	35	36	37	38	39	40	41	42	43	43	44	45	46	47	48	49	50
265	33	34	35	36	36	37	38	39	40	41	42	43	43	44	45	46	47	48	49
270	32	33	34	35	36	37	37	38	39	40	41	42	43	43	44	45	46	47	48
275	32	32	33	34	35	36	37	38	38	39	40	41	42	43	43	44	45	46	47
280	31	32	33	33	34	35	36	37	38	38	39	40	41	42	43	43	44	45	46
285	30	31	32	33	34	34	35	36	37	38	39	39	40	41	42	43	43	44	45
290	30	31	31	32	33	34	35	35	36	37	38	39	39	40	41	42	43	43	44
295	29	30	31	32	32	33	34	35	36	36	37	38	39	39	40	41	42	43	43
300	29	29	30	31	32	33	33	34	35	36	36	37	38	39	39	40	41	42	43

WORKSHEET—MEN

COMPUTING YOUR PERCENT BODY FAT

First, find your average measurements IN INCHES or POUNDS of:

	Wrist	Abdomen	Weight
measurement #1	____	____	____
+			
measurement #2	____	____	
+			
measurement #3	____	____	
total =	____	____	
divide by 3 =	____	____	

From your waist measurement _____

subtract your wrist measurement − _____

_____= "waist minus wrist"

Using Table 4.3, find your weight in pounds in the left-hand column. Find your "waist minus wrist" number across the top of the chart. Going across from the left and down from the top, find the point at which these two readings intersect. This figure represents your percent body fat.

From Table 4.3, _____ = percent body fat

at both extremes of your age range and subtract them each from 100. Divide the resulting numbers into your lean-body weight and multiply the result by 100. The figures you obtain will bracket your ideal body weight range. Let's look at an example:

A female, age 34
Lean-body weight 96 lbs (calculated as above)
Ideal body fat percentage from table 4.1 = 21–27%

Step 1: Subtract each of the ranges of ideal fat from 100.

100% − 21% = 79%   and   100% − 27% = 73%

Step 2: Divide lean body weight by these numbers.

96/79 = 1.22   and   96/73 = 1.32

Step 3: Multiply these numbers by 100.

1.22 × 100 = 122   and   1.32 × 100 = 132

This calculation gives an ideal body weight range of 122 to 132 pounds.

In this lady's case, given her lean-body weight, she should ideally and realistically weigh somewhere between 122 and 132 pounds. The figures in this example are actually those of one of my patients. She is 5'3" tall, and by the "ideal" weight charts, should weigh 115 pounds. Since reaching adulthood, she has never weighed 115 pounds and is not likely to, since at that weight, with her lean-body weight of 96 pounds, she would carry only about 16 percent body fat—an unhealthy proposition in a thirty-four-year-old woman.

I have provided space and instructions for these arithmetical maneuvers on your worksheet, but in case you have an aversion to mathematics, I have made it simpler still with yet another table, Table 4.4. On Table 4.4 you will find your lean body weight on the left side and your percentage body-fat goal across the top. At the intersection of a line drawn from your lean-body weight to the right, and from your body-fat goal down, you will find your goal weight.

IDEAL BODY WEIGHT
WORKSHEET

Your calculated lean-body weight = _____

Ideal body-fat range percentage for your age and sex from Table 4.1:

_____% to _____%

Step 1: Subtract each of these percents from 100:

100% − _____% = _____ and 100% − _____% = _____

Step 2: Divide your lean-body weight by each of the numbers from step 1:

_____ / _____ = _____ and _____ / _____ = _____

Step 3: Multiply each of these answers from step 2 by 100:

_____ × 100 = _____

your ideal weight is
in this range

_____ × 100 = _____

Let's look at a few examples from my practice to see some different applications of these computations.

Melissa M. . . . .

Melissa M. is a nineteen-year-old female college student who is active in intramural athletics. She is 5'4" tall and weighs 153 pounds. According to the "ideal" height/weight charts, Melissa should weigh around 120 pounds. Prior to coming to me, she had dieted twice—very rigidly—and had even increased her level of activity, but she was never able to get within 10 pounds of the "magic" 120-pound figure. What was her problem?

Her hip circumference was 41 inches, her waist, 30 inches. Checking on Table 4.2, we find her constants to be 48.84 for her hips, 21.33 for her waist, and 39.01 for her height of 64 inches.

$$
\begin{array}{rl}
\text{constant A} & 48.84 \\
\text{plus constant B} + & 21.33 \\
= & 70.17 \\
\text{minus constant C} - & 39.01 \\
= & 31.16 = 31\% \text{ body fat}
\end{array}
$$

31% body fat × 153 lbs (.31 × 153 = 47.4) = 47 lbs fat

153 lbs total weight − 47 lbs fat = 106 lbs lean-body weight

From table 4.1, we find that Melissa should carry between 20 and 26 percent body fat, not 31 percent. When we plug these values into Table 4.4, we find that Melissa, ideally, should weigh somewhere between 132.5 and 143 pounds. It's easy to see why Melissa had trouble reaching 120 pounds. At that weight, with her lean-body weight of 106 pounds, she would have carried only 11.5 percent body fat—an almost impossible proposition in all but the most athletic females.

Barbara L. . . . .

Barbara L. is a thirty-seven-year-old attorney who was the same height and weight as Melissa M.—5'4" tall, and 153 pounds. Her body size was, however, much different. Barbara's waist and hip measurements were 43 and 44 inches respectively. From Table 4.2 and the worksheet, we find that of Barbara's total weight, 38 percent

T A B L E   4 . 4

Goal Weight Calculations

Lean Body Weight	12	13	14	15	16	17	18	19	20	21	22	23	24	25	26	27	28	29	30	31
86	98	99	100	101	102	104	105	106	108	109	110	112	113	115	116	118	119	121	123	125
88	100	101	102	104	105	106	107	109	110	111	113	114	116	117	119	121	122	124	126	128
90	102	103	105	106	107	108	110	111	113	114	115	117	118	120	122	123	125	127	129	130
92	105	106	107	108	110	111	112	114	115	116	118	119	121	123	124	126	128	130	131	133
94	107	108	109	111	112	113	115	116	118	119	121	122	124	125	127	129	131	132	134	136
96	109	110	112	113	114	116	117	119	120	122	123	125	126	128	130	132	133	135	137	139
98	111	113	114	115	117	118	120	121	123	124	126	127	129	131	132	134	136	138	140	142
100	114	115	116	118	119	120	122	123	125	127	128	130	132	133	135	137	139	141	143	145
102	116	117	119	120	121	123	124	126	128	129	131	132	134	136	138	140	142	144	146	148
104	118	120	121	122	124	125	127	128	130	132	133	135	137	139	141	142	144	146	149	151
106	120	122	123	125	126	128	129	131	133	134	136	138	139	141	143	145	147	149	151	154
108	123	124	126	127	129	130	132	133	135	137	138	140	142	144	146	148	150	152	154	157
110	125	126	128	129	131	133	134	136	138	139	141	143	145	147	149	151	153	155	157	159
112	127	129	130	132	133	135	137	138	140	142	143	145	147	149	151	153	156	158	160	162
114	130	131	133	134	136	137	139	141	143	144	146	148	150	152	154	156	158	161	163	165
116	132	133	135	136	138	140	141	143	145	147	149	151	153	155	157	159	161	163	166	168
118	134	136	137	139	140	142	144	146	148	149	151	153	155	157	159	162	164	166	169	171

120	136	138	140	141	143	145	146	148	150	152	154	156	158	160	162	164	167	169	171	174
122	139	140	142	144	145	147	149	151	153	154	156	158	161	163	165	167	169	172	174	177
124	141	143	144	146	148	149	151	153	155	157	159	161	163	165	168	170	172	175	177	180
126	143	145	147	148	150	152	154	156	158	159	162	164	166	168	170	173	175	177	180	183
128	145	147	149	151	152	154	156	158	160	162	164	166	168	171	173	175	178	180	183	186
130	148	149	151	153	155	157	159	160	163	165	167	169	171	173	176	178	181	183	186	188
132	150	152	153	155	157	159	161	163	165	167	169	171	174	176	178	181	183	186	189	191
134	152	154	156	158	160	161	163	165	168	170	172	174	176	179	181	184	186	189	191	194
136	155	156	158	160	162	164	166	168	170	172	174	177	179	181	184	186	189	192	194	197
138	157	159	160	162	164	166	168	170	173	175	177	179	182	184	186	189	192	194	197	200
140	159	161	163	165	167	169	171	173	175	177	179	182	184	187	189	192	194	197	200	203
142	161	163	165	167	169	171	173	175	178	180	182	184	187	189	192	195	197	200	203	206
144	164	166	167	169	171	173	176	178	180	182	185	187	189	192	195	197	200	203	206	209
146	166	168	170	172	174	176	178	180	183	185	187	190	192	195	197	200	203	206	209	212
148	168	170	172	174	176	178	180	183	185	187	190	192	195	197	200	203	206	208	211	214
150	170	172	174	176	179	181	183	185	188	190	192	195	197	200	203	205	208	211	214	217
152	173	175	177	179	181	183	185	188	190	192	195	197	200	203	205	208	211	214	217	220
154	175	177	179	181	183	186	188	190	193	195	197	200	203	205	208	211	214	217	220	223
156	177	179	181	184	186	188	190	193	195	197	200	203	205	208	211	214	217	220	223	226
158	180	182	184	186	188	190	193	195	198	200	203	205	208	211	214	216	219	223	226	229
160	182	184	186	188	190	193	195	198	200	203	205	208	211	213	216	219	222	225	229	232
162	184	186	188	191	193	195	198	200	203	205	208	210	213	216	219	222	225	228	231	235
164	186	189	191	193	195	198	200	202	205	208	210	213	216	219	222	225	228	231	234	238
166	189	191	193	195	198	200	202	205	208	210	213	216	218	221	224	227	231	234	237	241

TABLE 4.4

Goal Weight Calculations

Lean Body Weight	12	13	14	15	16	17	18	19	20	21	22	23	24	25	26	27	28	29	30	31
168	191	193	195	198	200	202	205	207	210	213	215	218	221	224	227	230	233	237	240	243
170	193	195	198	200	202	205	207	210	213	215	218	221	224	227	230	233	236	239	243	246
172	195	198	200	202	205	207	210	212	215	218	221	223	226	229	232	236	239	242	246	249
174	198	200	202	205	207	210	212	215	218	220	223	226	229	232	235	238	242	245	249	252
176	200	202	205	207	210	212	215	217	220	223	226	229	232	235	238	241	244	248	251	255
178	202	205	207	209	212	214	217	220	223	225	228	231	234	237	241	244	247	251	254	258
180	205	207	209	212	214	217	220	222	225	228	231	234	237	240	243	247	250	254	257	261
182	207	209	212	214	217	219	222	225	228	230	233	236	239	243	246	249	253	256	260	264
184	209	211	214	216	219	222	224	227	230	233	236	239	242	245	249	252	256	259	263	267
186	211	214	216	219	221	224	227	230	233	235	238	242	245	248	251	255	258	262	266	270
188	214	216	219	221	224	227	229	232	235	238	241	244	247	251	254	258	261	265	269	272
190	216	218	221	224	226	229	232	235	238	241	244	247	250	253	257	260	264	268	271	275
192	218	221	223	226	229	231	234	237	240	243	246	249	253	256	259	263	267	270	274	278
194	220	223	226	228	231	234	237	240	243	246	249	252	255	259	262	266	269	273	277	281
196	223	225	228	231	233	236	239	242	245	248	251	255	258	261	265	268	272	276	280	284
198	225	228	230	233	236	239	241	244	248	251	254	257	261	264	268	271	275	279	283	287
200	227	230	233	235	238	241	244	247	250	253	256	260	263	267	270	274	278	282	286	290

202	230	232	235	238	240	243	246	249	253	256	259	262	266	269	273	277	281	285	289	293
204	232	234	237	240	243	246	249	252	255	258	262	265	268	272	276	279	283	287	291	296
206	234	237	240	242	245	248	251	254	258	261	264	268	271	275	278	282	286	290	294	299
208	236	239	242	245	248	251	254	257	260	263	267	270	274	277	281	285	289	293	297	301
210	239	241	244	247	250	253	256	259	263	266	269	273	276	280	284	288	292	296	300	304
212	241	244	247	249	252	255	259	262	265	268	272	275	279	283	286	290	294	299	303	307
214	243	246	249	252	255	258	261	264	268	271	274	278	282	285	289	293	297	301	306	310
216	245	248	251	254	257	260	263	267	270	273	277	281	284	288	292	296	300	304	309	313
218	248	251	253	256	260	263	266	269	273	276	279	283	287	291	295	299	303	307	311	316
220	250	253	256	259	262	265	268	272	275	278	282	286	289	293	297	301	306	310	314	319
222	252	255	258	261	264	267	271	274	278	281	285	288	292	296	300	304	308	313	317	322
224	255	257	260	264	267	270	273	277	280	284	288	291	295	299	303	307	311	315	320	325
226	257	260	263	266	269	272	276	279	283	286	290	294	297	301	305	310	314	318	323	328
228	259	262	265	268	271	275	278	281	285	289	292	296	300	304	308	312	317	321	326	330
230	261	264	267	271	274	277	280	284	288	291	295	299	303	307	311	315	319	324	329	333
232	264	267	270	273	276	280	283	286	290	294	297	301	305	309	314	318	322	327	331	336
234	266	269	272	275	279	282	285	289	293	296	300	304	308	312	316	321	325	330	334	339
236	268	271	274	278	281	284	288	291	295	299	303	306	311	315	319	323	328	332	337	342
238	270	274	277	280	283	287	290	294	298	301	305	309	313	317	322	326	331	335	340	345
240	273	276	279	282	286	289	293	296	300	304	308	312	316	320	324	329	333	338	343	348
242	275	278	281	285	288	292	295	299	303	306	310	314	318	323	327	332	336	341	346	351
244	277	280	284	287	290	294	298	301	305	309	313	317	321	325	330	334	339	344	349	354
246	280	283	286	289	293	296	300	304	308	311	315	319	324	328	332	337	342	346	351	357

is body fat—markedly different from Melissa's 31 percent although both are the same height and weight. Of her 153 pounds, 58 are fat, leaving a lean-body weight (LBW) of 95 pounds. With this LBW, we find from Table 4.4 that her goal weight should range from 120 to 130 pounds. Barbara can realistically reach the 120-pound goal recommended by the ideal height/weight tables.

These two examples illustrate why two people with exactly the same height and weight have different goal weights, and why the LBW determination methods are much more accurate and realistic than are various height/weight table calculations. The next patient has a problem, however, that can't be dealt with as easily as could Melissa's and Barbara's.

Joan F. . . . .

Joan F. came to my office weighing 250 pounds and suffering from a host of problems related to her obesity. She was forty-three years old and had been "heavy" all her life. Her height was, coincidentally, the same as Barbara's and Melissa's, 5'4", but her measurements were substantially different with her waist being 43 inches while her hips were 47 inches. We calculated her body fat to be 49 percent, her fat weight 125 pounds, and her LBW to be 125 pounds. The problem occurred when we calculated her goal weight based on this 125 pound LBW and found it to be in the 160 to 174 pound range—Joan wanted desperately to weigh no more than 140 pounds. At 140 pounds, with a 125 pound LBW, she would have only about 10 percent body fat—a near impossibility with her age and level of activity. Is Joan doomed to never go below 160 pounds? Not necessarily.

If Joan loses down to 160 pounds on the PSMF, she will have lost 95 pounds. She has, through the years, increased her LBW to support this extra weight, and as she loses weight overall, she will lose some of this excess LBW. In some instances, very obese patients lose up to 20 percent of their LBW as their weight decreases on the PSMF. Assuming Joan's LBW diminishes by only 12 percent to 110 pounds, if she attains a 22 percent body-fat level—the bottom range for her age—she would weigh 141 pounds.

Walt H. . . . .

Let's see how these calculations work with men. Walt H. is thirty-eight years old, weighs 230 pounds, and wants to lose "about twenty pounds." His height, 6'1", is of no consequence to us since height—by this method—does not figure into body fat determination for men. His waist circumference is 45.5 inches and his wrist measures 7.5 inches around.

$$\text{waist (45.5)} - \text{wrist (7.5)} = 38$$

From Table 4.3 we find that at 230 pounds and with a waist-minus-wrist measurement of 38, Walt carries 33 percent body fat, and by calculation, has a LBW of 154 pounds. Table 4.1 shows that his body fat should be in the 13 to 19 percent range, and by turning to Table 4.4 we can see that his goal weight should be in the 177 to 190 pound range—requiring a loss of 40 to 53 pounds.

When I showed Walt these calculations and proposed that he undertake the PSMF to reach his goal weight range, he was hesitant about losing that much weight. He thought that he would appear "skinny" at that lower weight because he had weighed 210 pounds when he played college football and thought that he "looked great then." He didn't want to lose much below that.

His reluctance brings up a problem that I often encounter in my practice. Men almost always suppose that they should weigh the same as they did when they were in their late teens or early twenties. They think that if they can just weigh what they did in college, they will have the same physique they had then and even be able to wear the same size clothing. In almost all situations, this is not the case. As men age and become less active, they lose some of the muscle mass they previously had. This usually happens at the same time that they are gaining scale weight, which means that in addition to merely gaining extra fat, they are also replacing muscle with fat. This is exactly what happened in Walt's case. He told me that when he weighed 210 pounds in college, he had a 33-inch waist. If we assume that his wrist diameter was the same then as it is now—7.5 inches—then his waist-minus-wrist measurement would have been 25.5. From Table 4.3 we find that Walt had 8 percent body fat while weighing 210 pounds eighteen years earlier—about right for a young, heavily muscled athlete in excellent physical condition. His LBW was 193 pounds—almost 40 pounds more than the 154 pound LBW he has now. If he were to lose only to 210 pounds while maintaining his 154-pound LBW, he would be carrying 56 pounds or almost 27 percent body fat. This is considerably more than the 13 to 19 percent he should be carrying, and substantially more than the 8 percent he carried while in college. Unless Walt has plans—which he doesn't—of returning to the level of activity he maintained while in college, he can't expect to maintain the same physique. In order for him to be slim and carry the appropriate amount of body fat, he must weigh less than he did in college. Fortunately, I was able—by the use of these tables—to convince Walt of the logic of this argument, and he went on to lose the required amount of weight on the PSMF, and he has maintained his lower weight.

Fat Distribution Patterns

If you determine from the tables and worksheets that you are carrying an extra thirty pounds of fat, does it matter where this fat is located? Does it make a difference if it is on your hips, legs, or abdominal area? Does fat come off faster with dieting if it is hip fat versus abdominal fat? Fat location is indeed significant—and very important in terms of health.

The two basic types of fat distribution—android and gynoid—are, for the most part, a function of the sex of the individual in question, with females usually having the gynoid type, males the android. Males can, however, have a gynoid fat distribution and females can have an android distribution, but generally this is not the case.

The *gynoid* fat distribution pattern is classically the "pear" shaped configuration, with most of the fat being carried on the hips and upper legs. These are not the only places excess fat is carried, but they are the areas where additional fat is first deposited. And since fat comes off in the same order in which it went on, the legs and hips are the last places to lose during a diet. As women (or anyone with a gynoid fat pattern) gain fat, it is deposited first on their hips and upper legs, and then on their abdomen, arms, face, and neck, and the rest of their body in general, but the same basic ratios apply: their hips gain more, faster, than anywhere else. The gynoid pattern of fat distribution carries relatively less health risk than does the android.

The *android* fat distribution, in fruit terms, would be the "apple" shaped body. Here, most of the fat is carried on the abdominal area. People who have "beer bellies," with smaller hips and upper bodies, have the android fat pattern. As is the case with the gynoid pattern, fat is first deposited on the waist and then to a lesser extent on other areas, and during dieting, it comes off in reverse order. The android fat distribution pattern poses substantial health risks.

Based on estimates from my practice, probably 70 percent of women have a pure gynoid fat pattern, while 30 percent have an android or mixed pattern. Males, on the other hand, almost always have an android pattern. Occasionally, I see a man with a gynoid fat distribution, but very infrequently—maybe 1–2 percent of male patients.

To determine your type of fat distribution, you must measure your waist at the umbilicus and your hips at their widest point. Divide your waist measurement by your hip measurement and find the resultant figure—your waist-to-hip ratio—in Table 4.5.

The figures in Table 4.5 are approximations. If you are female, and your waist-to-hip ratio is 0.84, it doesn't necessarily mean that you have a pure android fat distribution pattern, only that you tend in that direction more than someone with a ratio of 0.76. The same holds true in reverse for males with a ratio of less than 1.

Once you have determined your waist-to-hip ratio, what does this tell you—other than where your fat is located—about your ability to lose weight, or your disease-risk profile? As you might suspect, there are variations on both as a function of fat-pattern distribution type.

I have seen one study, comparing the rate of weight loss with waist-to-hip ratio, that seemed to indicate that there was no significant difference in the rapidity of weight loss as a function of body fat distribution. My own experience, however, does not bear this out.

T A B L E 4.5

Waist-to-Hip Ratios

Males	less than 1: gynoid 1 or greater: android
Females	0.8 or less: gynoid greater than 0.8: android

I have found that patients with an android fat pattern typically lose weight at a more rapid rate than do patients with a gynoid pattern. This is not true just because they are usually males, as women that I treat who have an android pattern also routinely lose at a faster rate. In addition, it seems that excess fat other than the fat in the pure gynoid distribution comes off more rapidly. Women—and men with a gynoid pattern—lose fat from their arms, necks, abdomens, and backs at a fairly rapid rate, but the remaining hip and upper-leg fat recedes more slowly. In fact, this time between the rapid loss of upper-body fat and the slower loss of lower-body fat is the critical point at which many women abandon their diets. They have become accustomed to routinely losing several pounds per week, and when this rate decreases because they have lost down to solely the pure excess gynoid fat, which for unknown reasons hangs on tenaciously, they despair, become discouraged, and often quit. You must remain aware of this danger point and understand that the lower-body fat absolutely *will* come off, but only if you adhere to your regimen.

Those with a gynoid fat distribution should find some comfort in the fact that theirs is a relatively healthy fat. Many more people with excess lower-body fat live to an advanced age, with fewer health problems as a result of their fat, than do people with large abdominal girths. Try to remember aged people that you have known. You will find that you can probably recall many very elderly women with large hips and legs, but not many very elderly men with large abdomens. The fat pattern difference is no doubt one of the reasons for the divergence between males and females on the mortality charts. As the waist-to-hip ratio of males increases above 1, the risk of these diseases increases proportionately. The same holds true for females as the waist-to-hip ratio increases beyond 0.8.

Abdominal fat is associated with an increased risk of hypertension (high blood pressure), diabetes, and heart disease, which are not so strongly associated with lower-body fat. The increased risk arises because the blood circulating through abdominal fat empties—via large blood vessels—directly into the liver, causing metabolic derangements. Fluids from lower-body fat are generally transported through the lymphatic system and through other round-about ways to the liver, giving them time to become much more dilute, and consequently much less demanding upon the metabolic capacities of the liver. But please understand that while individuals who carry their fat primarily in the "lower body" have a lesser health risk than those who carry their fat around the abdomen, they still have a greater health risk than those with a normal amount of lower-body fat. Making the effort to lose surplus fat from all areas is a small premium to pay for the dividends of better health and an improved appearance.

Erratic Weight Loss

There is nothing more disappointing to both doctor and patient alike than a tiny or even no weight loss after a week of meticulous adherence to a dietary regimen. Unfortunately, this can happen even on the PSMF. Patients sometimes come into the clinic radiantly happy, exclaiming that they feel terrific and that all their clothing is now hanging loosely on them, that they have been human dynamos the previous week and have accomplished countless tasks; then they step on the scales. If they have not lost some preconceived amount of weight, they despair and within moments go from being wildly ebullient to being disheartened and discouraged. You would think that it would be obvious if their clothing is much looser that they were decreasing in size, but they oftentimes don't see it that way—they are fixated on weight. In an effort to keep this from happening to you, let's look at another model of what comprises weight.

This is a different model than that which we looked at previously, but it should help you better understand what you do and do not have control over with regard to weight loss. (Lest you think they are simplistic, these types of diagrammatic models of the body are routinely used in the training of medical students to demonstrate different physiological characteristics.) In the average person, about 15 percent of the body weight is composed of fat, 25 percent is protein, mineral, and related substances, and the rest—about 60 percent—is water. Of this 60 percent that is water, 40 percent is water inside the cells of the body, and 20 percent is the water outside the cells. When we looked at our earlier model that was just fat and lean, we included the water weight of both these tissues. In the model below, we have broken out the portion of weight contributed separately by the water content of both fat and lean.

PROTEIN 25%	WATER 60%	FAT 15%

Let's take a look at what we can actually control with dieting. We can reduce our fat by limiting our caloric intake and by exercise—which is great. We can reduce our lean tissue weight by consuming inadequate amounts of protein and by not exercising—which is not so good. What can we do about our water weight? Nothing, really. We can't influence the amount of water that goes into or comes out of the cell; we can't make ourselves have less or more blood. Without the use of medications, the effects of which are only temporary, we have no control over the amount of water in our bodies—yet this water represents 60 percent of our weight.

The human body has a multitude of physiological feedback mechanisms—many hormonal—that dictate the amount and distribution of body water. Many people take diuretics (water pills)—never recommended for weight loss—and artificially cause their bodies to release some water as urine, but as soon as they quit taking the medicine, the water comes back. Women have menstrual cycles that influence the amount of body water they retain. The consumption of alcohol and carbohydrates affects the amount of body water we retain, and these we can restrict, but their influence represents only a small amount of the body water gained or lost. For the most part, the amount of body water we maintain is regulated by factors completely beyond our control.

It is easy to see how small increases in the water compartment of our body—due to hormonal variation, heat, or a multitude of causes—can offset fairly large losses of fat. This is particularly true since fat is lighter on a volume basis than is water—a glass of water would weigh about 11 percent more than the same glass filled with fat. Butter, lard, and other fats and oils float on water because of this density difference, and for this same reason, slender, muscular people sink in swimming pools while obese people float.

The point of all this is that you shouldn't worry if occasionally you don't seem to be losing weight. If you are following the PSMF regimen properly, you *will* be losing fat, and that is what counts.

Fat weighs about 7.5 pounds per gallon, so if you lose 3.5 pounds of fat in one week, you have lost almost half a gallon of volume (or size). By the same token, if you weigh 150 pounds, 90 of these pounds are water, and just a 3 percent change in the amount of water you are carrying—for whatever reason—will offset the loss of over two pounds of fat. But you will still decrease in size, and in percent body fat, and that is what matters.

I encourage my patients to put on an article of clothing—usually a pair of slacks—that they cannot get into comfortably, then remove the clothing and weigh. After one week, they are to try the slacks on again and notice how much more comfortably they fit. Then they weigh, and if they have sustained a good weight loss, wonderful; but if they haven't, it doesn't matter because it is obvious that they are losing fat. I recommend that you follow this same procedure and let the weight—over which you have little control —take care of itself. When you finish the PSMF and divide the amount of time you spent adhering to it into the total amount of weight you lost, you will find that you lost somewhere from 2 to 5 pounds per week. So, *don't* let your mood or hopes rise or fall depending upon the amount of weight you lose—or fail to lose— in any given week. Concentrate instead on those things over which you have control.

5

Losing Fat
on the PSMF

*T*HE regimen I use in my practice consists of three phases—
the weight-loss phase, the transitional phase, and finally, the
maintenance phase. I want you to see how these phases all
fit together forming the total dietary plan, and then, in a chapter
devoted to each, we will examine each phase separately.

Weight-Loss Phase

The first phase of any diet—and unfortunately, the only phase
for many dieters—is the weight-loss phase. It is here that you get
rid of most of your excess fat while undergoing the most stringent
part of the regimen. It is also the easiest of any part of a long-term
weight-reduction plan to follow: your motivation is high and you
lose large amounts of weight and size quickly. During this phase,
you will use the PSMF *exactly* as described in Chapter 6 as your
weight-loss tool. Your modified fasting regimen will consist of four
high-protein supplements and one protein meal daily, the specifics
of which are detailed in the next chapter. You should remain on
this modified fasting program until you are very near your goal
weight. If your doctor provides your supplement during this phase,

you may remain solely on these supplements without the protein meal I recommend until you reach your goal. If you are preparing your own supplements, however, it is absolutely *essential* that you follow the regimen *exactly* as it is described in the next chapter.

If followed correctly, this weight-loss phase should result in your losing from 2 to 5 pounds per week, a decrease in your blood pressure, an improvement in most "sugar" metabolism problems you might have, and a lowering—often substantial—of your serum cholesterol and triglycerides. You should experience all these beneficial effects while remaining hunger free and having an increased level of energy. You also will find that you will accomplish much more than usual because you will not spend as much time eating or being involved in activities related to food. If you are like most patients who have been on this regimen, you will be reluctant to move on to the next phase because you will have found the PSMF to have been simple to follow, and yet quite satisfying.

Transitional Phase

In this second phase, described in Chapter 7, you will start back on the road to regular food. As you come off the PSMF, you will first eat foods that have approximately the same proportions of protein and carbohydrate as the PSMF. You will then gradually increase the amount of carbohydrate in your diet until you reach your maintenance level. While in the transitional phase, you should continue to lose weight, but not at quite the same rate as during the PSMF. For this reason, you should start the transitional phase when you are from 3 to 7 pounds from your goal weight.

The very first part of the transitional phase diet also serves another purpose: it acts as a "recovery" diet. No matter how diligently you may try to adhere to any dietary maintenance plan, there will be times when you overindulge. These culinary transgressions are the undoing of most dieters, but you can overcome them. The secret is judicious use of the recovery diet. It is unrealistic for me to expect you—or for you to expect yourself, for that matter—to go on a maintenance program, irrespective of how good it is, and never veer from it. Knowing this, it makes sense to have a plan to turn to when the inevitable happens. If you have a long weekend "blowout," you can follow it with the transitional phase meals for two days and almost always rid yourself of the excess weight you picked up. We will discuss this "recovery" diet in detail in a later chapter.

Maintenance

The maintenance phase of any diet is, without question, the most difficult to adhere to. Practically everyone who is now overweight has lost weight at some time but unfortunately has put it back on. The so-called yo-yo syndrome is widespread among dieters. It is frustrating and discouraging to endure a lengthy diet, lose to your goal weight, and then inexorably gain it all back. Part of the problem is that most dieters think of only the weight-loss phase when they think of dieting. They seem to believe that there is something magical about attaining a goal weight, and that once there, they are dietarily invincible. For most dieters, attaining their goal weight becomes the end point of their diet, when in fact, it should be only the beginning. Don't make it your plan to diet until you reach 120 pounds or 135 pounds or 170 pounds or whatever goal weight you may have in mind; plan instead to *remain* at that goal weight for five years—*that* should be your goal. If all you plan to do is reach a certain goal weight and then regain to where you are now—don't bother. Why waste your time, why deprive yourself when it's all for nothing? It's not worth the effort to get to 125 pounds just to stay there for one month. Just recognize that you're overweight, quit worrying about it, don't waste your money on weight-loss programs, and get on with your life. But if you want to *stay* at your goal weight and retain the lower blood pressure, the lower blood cholesterol, and all the other health benefits you have worked for, then you must maintain, maintain, maintain.

The maintenance phase I will offer in Chapter 8 is a *realistic* diet plan that you can remain on for the rest of your life. It allows you to eat anything and everything you want, as long as you follow the diet protocols *most* of the time. You will use the maintenance plan I've outlined as your dietary baseline to which you will return after occasional episodes of overindulgence followed by recovery. Since the basic maintenance plan does not include many foods with a high carbohydrate content such as candy, pastries, french fries, malted milk, pancakes, and many others, you must either give them up forever—a difficult proposition if you really love or crave these foods—or modify the regimen so that it allows you to have them without gaining weight. The choice of forsaking these foods forever, no matter how well intentioned, is not realistic. You won't be able to do it. But if you do try to adopt this hard-line approach, the moment you succumb to the temptation of, for example, a cheese Danish, you will lose a little self-esteem, and the idea will become implanted a little more firmly that you can't stay on a diet. It is much more realistic to remain on the maintenance diet the majority of the time, allowing yourself periodic dietary vacations that you *plan* for and enjoy without guilt, and then recover from them. *The secret is in the recovery.*

The actual basic maintenance diet is far from limited. It is a low-carbohydrate/high-protein regimen made of meat, fish, cheese, eggs, salads, fruits, fresh vegetables, butter, mayonnaise, bread, specially made desserts, and even fast foods such as pizza, hamburgers, and fajitas. With this varied menu, you won't need to take your dietary vacations very often, but it's nice to know that they are available when you need them. Most of the time, however, you will stay on the maintenance menus, which are very satisfying and surprisingly easy to prepare, and which allow you to retain the health benefits you achieved on the PSMF.

On the program I have developed, you will start by determining your realistic ideal weight, percentage body fat goal, and the amount of fat you need to lose to attain this. You will then begin with the PSMF, which is easy to follow and produces rapid and substantial fat loss. As you approach your ideal weight, you will progress to the transition phase, which allows you to ease off the PSMF and onto the maintenance phase, while continuing to lose the last few pounds. The maintenance phase, which you adapt to your own culinary preferences, will be your lifelong blueprint for health and thinness.

Getting Started

By now I hope you're sold on the idea of losing large amounts of body fat rapidly and without staying hungry. You've seen an overview of the program from the weight-loss phase through maintenance, so let's get started. The first thing you should do is to inform your physician that you are planning to embark on this regimen. He or she may provide the supplements for you, do your baseline lab and EKG studies, and monitor your progress—or may refer you to a physician who is experienced in the use of the PSMF. If you have no physician, you may find one by following the instructions as outlined in Appendix A, "How to Find a Doctor."

The modified version of the PSMF described in this book is safe if followed *exactly* as instructed, but you should nevertheless consult with your physician to make sure that you are in good health and have no underlying problems that are causing you to be overweight, or that could be made worse by the PSMF. Along with a physical exam, you should have the following studies done: an EKG, a complete blood count, a blood chemistry panel including electrolytes, a urinalysis, and a blood cholesterol test that detects the amounts of the various cholesterol subunits. These studies will provide you and your physician with a picture of your current health to be used as a baseline and compared with lab results obtained during the course of the PSMF.[1]

Can Anyone Go on the PSMF?

Unfortunately, good as it is, the PSMF is not for everyone. Some people, because of certain underlying health problems, are not good candidates for the PSMF. The criteria listed below were those in use when this book was written, in late 1988, and may change. As physicians accumulate more experience in the use of the PSMF, some will feel more secure in trying higher-risk patients on the regimen and will publish their experiences for the benefit of all physicians; perhaps then the criteria will change. At first, obese children and adolescents were excluded from the program because physicians thought that the very low calorie and carbohydrate intake would interfere with normal growth. Then, after a careful study of several groups of adolescents who were monitored closely and found to have no growth problems, the criteria were changed to allow adolescents to undertake the PSMF. So, if you find yourself listed

---

[1]Most of the expense involved with the PSMF is due to the many lab tests required. Fortunately, many, if not most, of these costs can be recouped from your insurance company if you have health insurance. An increasing number of insurance companies are becoming more enlightened about the fact that obesity is a disease and consequently are reimbursing for the PSMF. A large portion of this acceptance is due to the astounding results patients have obtained by using the PSMF. Since overweight people have many more serious health problems than do normal weight people, it makes sense from the insurance industry's perspective to pay a little now to help these people improve their health rather than pay much more later to treat the medical problems caused by their obesity.

in the categories below, discuss your situation with your physician: it may be possible for him or her to modify the program in a way that will not put you at risk, or perhaps the criteria will have changed by the time you read this and you will have been found to no longer be in a high-risk group.

First, let's look at the *absolute contraindications* to going on the PSMF as they now stand. People with the following conditions should *under no circumstances* undertake the PSMF:

1. Pregnancy or breast-feeding

2. Severe liver disease

3. Renal failure

4. Myocardial infarction (heart attack) within three months

5. Unstable angina

6. Cancer

7. Severe depression

8. Lithium use

9. Drug or alcohol abuse

10. Unstable cerebrovascular disease (recent stroke)

11. Prolonged Q-T interval (specific EKG change)

12. "Brittle" type I diabetes mellitus

13. Chronic high-dose steroid use

14. Bleeding peptic ulcer

There are some conditions that don't pose as great a risk as those mentioned above to going on the PSMF. These conditions, considered *relative contraindications,* are listed below:

1. Over age seventy

2. Certain arrhythmias

3. History of liver or kidney disease

4. History of transient ischemic attacks (pre-stroke condition)

5. Stable type I diabetes mellitus

Having any of these last five conditions does not totally eliminate you as a candidate for the PSMF, but it does mean that your
physician must make the decision about your participation and be
willing to supervise you *very* closely.

The formulation I provide in the following chapter has powdered milk as a major ingredient. Patients with a lactose intolerance
problem will need to obtain supplements from their physician or
substitute a powdered soy "milk" in place of the powdered cow's
milk.

If you have none of the above conditions and are in good health,
you should be able to start on the weight-loss phase of the modified
PSMF outlined in this book as soon as you are ready. If your doctor
does not supply the supplements but is willing to monitor you periodically, you can prepare your own supplements using the instructions in the next chapter.

6

The Weight-Loss Phase

*A*T this point, you are ready to go. You have had your physical exam, you have calculated your lean-body weight and your percentage body fat, and you have a realistic goal weight in mind. You are now ready to start on the weight-loss phase—a modified version of the Protein-Sparing Modified Fast. In this chapter, you will learn how to make the protein supplements, and how to prepare them in different ways to provide variety. You will learn what vitamins to add to your daily regimen and the importance of adequate fluid intake. In all, there are five essential components of the weight-loss phase, with a section of this chapter devoted to each:

- protein supplements: 4 per day
- protein-rich meal: 1 per day
- vitamin supplements: daily
- fluids: minimum of 64 ounces daily
- exercise: 3 to 5 times per week

Once you get the materials, prepare your supplements, and get started, you should remain on the PSMF until your weight approaches your ideal body weight as determined by the calculations you learned in Chapter 4. At that point, you will start the transition diet described in the next chapter, and then ultimately you will go on the maintenance regimen discussed in Chapter 8.

The diet formulated for the weight-loss phase of my program is low in calories yet constructed in a way that prevents the loss of lean-body mass. This regimen provides all the essential vitamins, minerals, and other nutrients in amounts that equal or exceed the U.S. RDAs. The modified version of the PSMF presented here provides approximately 1,000 calories per day and is adequate in all necessary nutrients—most of which come from food sources.

In this chapter I will instruct you in the preparation of these supplements and meals and will provide you with the specific vitamin, fluid, and exercise regimen to follow that will allow you to lose large amounts of *fat* quickly and safely. To insure your safety, follow this regimen *exactly* as described.

Preparing the Supplements

You will need several ingredients that can be purchased from most grocery and/or health food stores to prepare the basic supplement powder. Once you have done so, you can vary it in several ways to accommodate your own particular tastes. I have listed mailorder sources in Appendix B for those who cannot find the necessary ingredients in their area.

Basic Supplement Powder

Mix well:
  1 envelope nonfat dry milk powder (or enough powder to make one quart)
  4 tablespoons protein powder (approx. 8 grams per tbsp)*
  1 teaspoon granular fructose
  1 teaspoon NoSalt salt substitute or Morton's salt substitute†
Store the mix dry in an airtight container or plastic zip-closure bag.

This recipe makes four servings of supplement powder—enough for one day of modified fasting. I recommend preparing enough for a week at a time.

One serving supplement = 4 tbsp Basic Supplement Powder, reconstituted with 8–12 ounces of a sugar-free liquid such as

*See description of protein powder below.
†It is vital that this ingredient always be included.

water, Diet Coke (or any other diet soft drink), coffee, or others (see recipes listed below).

Choosing a Protein Powder

In most cities and towns, you will be able to find a health food or nutrition store. You may never have frequented such an establishment, but I can assure you from my own reconnaissance, they are there, and their shelves are crowded with protein powders of every description. With so many product choices, which powder is right? The answer is, many of them. You need only know what to look for on the label, and I have devoted this section to making certain that you will. The critical qualities to look for are:

1. *Complete protein:* High-quality protein supplement powders may be made from egg albumin (egg-white protein), calcium caseinate and lactalbumin (milk-solid proteins), or soybean powder. You must be certain that the powder you purchase contains all nine essential amino acids. If the product is made from egg or milk or a mixture of these, you can be assured that it contains all the essential amino acids. People with known allergies or intolerance to milk or egg can use the soy protein powders in their supplements, as these are also complete. Later in the chapter, I have listed a number of specific products by brand name, all of which are satisfactory protein sources.

2. *Contains NO sugar, starches, or carbohydrates:* Many protein powders have huge amounts of added carbohydrate, and use of such a product would—as you have learned in earlier chapters—defeat the purpose of a protein-sparing regimen.

3. *Protein concentration:* The amount of protein provided per serving should be listed on the back of most powdered protein products. This amount will vary from one product to the next; for example, one may contain 24 grams of protein in three heaping tablespoons, and the next may contain 18 grams in one tablespoon. The variance is not critical to your selection of a particular product, but you will need to take note of how many grams of protein your powder contains. *Each serving of Basic Supplement Powder should contain approximately 8 grams of complete protein.* The actual number of tablespoons that you will use to formulate your own supplement will depend entirely upon how many grams of protein per tablespoon your product contains. The calculation necessary to determine

this amount is quite simple: divide the grams of protein per serving (listed on the label) by the number of tablespoons per serving.

In our 24-gram example above, that would be:

24 grams per serving/3 tbsp per serving = 8 grams per tbsp

The powders also vary widely both in flavor (I have seen chocolate, vanilla, and strawberry) and smoothness of mixing from one product line to the next. With vanilla, you can create a nearly endless variety of flavors depending on which sugar-free mixer (diet soda, Crystal Light, Sugar-Free Kool-Aid, etc.) you select. Whether a particular product "tastes good" or doesn't—as I have learned by trying many of them, myself—rests entirely in the tastebuds of the dieter. Several times I have found a product that I thought tasted delicious, have brought it home to let my wife try it, and have been rewarded for my efforts with a grimace and a shudder and a "Yuck!" Lest you jump to the conclusion that my wife is the finicky one in the family, let me assure you that this same scenario has been played out in reverse with the same results. Once you are certain that the product you intend to purchase fulfills all the requirements listed above, I encourage you to pick a protein powder that tastes good to *you*.

Commercially Available Protein Powders

I have investigated the following specific products and have found them to be complete proteins. This listing is by no means complete—there are many other fine products available. Let me point out that on many, you will read in fine print on the labels: "Use as a food supplement only. Do not use for weight reduction." Isn't the whole point of going on the PSMF weight reduction? Yes, but we don't intend to rely upon these supplemental proteins for our entire dietary intake. We will use them as supplements. Used as such, they are perfectly safe, but since the "liquid protein" disaster (detailed in Chapter 2), many protein powders carry this labeling, regardless of their safety. Even though these products represent sources of complete protein, DO NOT use them in any manner except *exactly* as outlined in this book—as supplements on this regimen.

Please also note that there may be recipes or serving suggestions on the labels. Ignore these. Virtually all of these recipes contain far more carbohydrate than is permissible in the weight-loss phase of the modified PSMF. Use the powders only as a source of supplemental protein.

MLO Products
Available at a multitude of health and nutrition stores across the country and by mail (see Appendix B for address and toll-free number).

Instant Milk and Egg Protein—
    Concentration: 12 grams protein per tablespoon
    Carbohydrates: 0 grams per tablespoon
    Calories: 50 per tablespoon

Joe Weider Products
Available at a multitude of health and nutrition stores across the country and by mail (see Appendix B for address and toll-free number).

90-Plus Sugar-Free Milk, Egg, Amino, and Fiber—
    Concentration: 8 grams protein per tablespoon
    Carbohydrates: 0 grams per tablespoon
    Calories: 33 per tablespoon

Other Products
Check your local health and nutrition stores, or refer to Appendix B for available mail/phone information.

Plus Formula 398 Complete Protein Powder—
    Concentration: 13 grams protein per tablespoon
    Carbohydrates: 0 grams per tablespoon
    Calories: 50 per tablespoon
  Lewis Laboratories RDA—
    Concentration: 15 grams protein per tablespoon
    Carbohydrates: 2.5 grams per tablespoon
    Calories: 55 per tablespoon
  Sportstar High-Performance Protein Milk & Egg Blend
    Concentration: 13.5 grams protein per tablespoon
    Carbohydrates: Less than 1 gram per tablespoon
    Calories: 57 per tablespoon

Challenge Products
Available at General Nutrition Centers across the country or by
mail (see Appendix B for a national address).

Body Builder's Protein—
    Concentration: 12 grams protein per tablespoon
    Carbohydrates: Less than 1 gram per tablespoon
    Calories: 50 per tablespoon
Milk and Egg Protein—
    Concentration: 12 grams protein per tablespoon
    Carbohydrates: Less than 1 gram per tablespoon
    Calories: 55 per tablespoon
95% Isolated Soy Protein—
    Concentration: 8 grams protein per tablespoon
    Carbohydrates: 0 grams per tablespoon
    Calories: 33 per tablespoon

Mixing the Supplements

To make a single serving, add four level tablespoons of Basic
Supplement Powder to 8–12 ounces of very cold liquid and blend
in a blender or shake well in a jar with a tight-fitting lid (this caveat
is especially important when using carbonated beverages). Remember, use ONLY sugar-free and carbohydrate-free beverages, water,
or coffee to mix the supplements. Never use vegetable or fruit juices
or nondiet sodas, all of which contain large amounts of carbohydrate
(sugar).

Only your creativity limits the taste possibilities available to
you, thanks to the wide variety of diet sodas, sugar-free punches
and lemonades, and flavoring extracts currently on the market. To
help you get started, I have included a number of clinic-tested supplement drink variations developed by my patients and staff for the
PSMF program I use in my own practice. In these recipes, four level
tablespoons of Basic Supplement Powder equals "1 serving."

Chocoholic Delight

1 serving Basic Supplement Powder
1 12-oz can Faygo or Canfield's Diet Chocolate Soda (or any diet
        chocolate soda)

3–5 drops chocolate extract (or to taste)
Blend cold soda with dry ingredients and extract. Add crushed ice
and continue to blend to desired thickness.

Orange Blossom Special

1 serving Basic Supplement Powder
1 12-oz can diet orange soda (NO fruit juice added)
A dash of cinnamon or allspice
Blend cold soda with dry ingredients. Add crushed ice and continue
to blend to desired thickness.

Strawberry Blush

1 serving Basic Supplement Powder
1 12-oz can diet strawberry soda
3–5 drops rum extract (or to taste)
Blend cold soda with dry ingredients and extract. Add crushed ice
and continue to blend to desired thickness.

Lemon Meringue

1 serving Basic Supplement Powder
8 oz Crystal Light or Country Time Sugar-Free Lemonade
Shake or blend cold lemonade with dry powder.

Mocha Mint

1 serving Basic Supplement Powder
8 oz hot coffee (not boiling, just off warmer)
1 packet Equal or Sweet'N Low sweetener
3–5 drops each mint and chocolate extracts (or to taste)
Blend coffee with dry ingredients and extracts. Serve warm in the
cold weather for a nice change from a slush. This recipe can
also be made with cold coffee and ice for summer.

Rum 'n' Coke

1 serving Basic Supplement Powder
1 12-oz can Diet Coke or other diet cola
3–5 drops rum extract (or to taste)
Blend cold soda with dry ingredients and extract. Add crushed ice
and blend to desired thickness.

Almond Café au Lait

1 serving Basic Supplement Powder
8 oz hot or cold coffee
1 packet Equal or Sweet'N Low sweetener
3–5 drops almond extract (or to taste)
Blend hot coffee with dry ingredients and extract. Serve warm. For
iced almond coffee, use cold coffee, add ice, and blend to desired
thickness.

These recipes should get you started on the road to creativity,
but good taste doesn't necessarily demand that you go to any
culinary extremes. The supplement powder mixes well with any of
the carbohydrate-free diet beverages on the market today—just suit
your own taste. I have used Diet Dr Pepper, Diet Sprite or 7-Up,
Diet Cherry 7-Up, diet root beer, and have enjoyed them all. If you
are like most of my patients, you will soon hit upon a combination
that pleases you and will probably stick with it most of the time.

Protein Meal

Along with the four supplements you consume daily, you *must*
eat a protein meal. (If you are using a commercially prepared supplement such as Optifast, you may—at your physician's discretion
and under his supervision—consume five supplements daily without a meal; otherwise you *must* eat the meal.) This meal, along with
a daily vitamin supplement, will provide you with all the nutrients
necessary to maintain good health. The protein meal consists of:

6 ounces (cooked weight) of lean meat or fish
1 cup salad
1 cup vegetable

Meat: Lean beef, pork, or lamb, baked, grilled, or broiled, with all visible fat trimmed before cooking; fish of any description as long as it is broiled, baked, or grilled with *no* breading or batter; or chicken without the skin, baked, broiled, or grilled, but with no breading or batter. It's acceptable to use *small* amounts of seasoning sauces such as Worcestershire sauce, or even *occasionally* the Mr. Ron's Barbecue Sauce (see recipe in Chapter 9), but don't overdo it during the weight-loss phase.

Salad: One cup loosely packed lettuce of any type with no more than one-quarter of a medium tomato. You may add *small* amounts of onion, mushroom, radishes, or cucumber for taste, but reduce the lettuce by an equal amount so that when prepared, your salad is approximately one cup in volume. Any commercially prepared vinegar and oil salad dressing (that has little or no carbohydrate) or the salad dressings listed in Chapter 9 are allowable in 2–3 tablespoon amounts. Lemon juice and plain vinegar and oil are also permitted.

Vegetable: One cup *raw* volume of a vegetable completes the meal. The following vegetables may be either steamed, baked, boiled, or eaten raw: broccoli, zucchini, asparagus, brussels sprouts, or cauliflower.

It is acceptable to occasionally have two cups of salad instead of salad and vegetable, or have two cups of vegetable instead of salad, but try as often as possible to adhere to the regimen as outlined.

Patients always ask me if it makes a difference what time of day this meal is eaten. Is it better to eat it for lunch or for supper? Since many studies have shown that people can lose weight by shifting more of their caloric intake to earlier in the day, it would seem prudent to eat the meal early in the day rather than late, but I don't think it really matters a great deal. Since it is the only meal eaten, most people prefer to eat it as the evening meal with their families. We will discuss some variations of this later on in the chapter.

Vitamin Supplementation

Many of the protein powders that are available are fortified with extra vitamins and minerals in addition to the ones found in the eggs, milk solids, and/or soybean powder, and combined with the protein meal, they will provide you with a level of nutrient intake that is adequate in all categories as defined in the RDAs. But to insure that these requirements are all met, I recommend that you take a multivitamin supplement daily. There are several good brands to choose from listed below. If none of these is available in your area, you might ask your physician or pharmacist to recommend something comparable. It probably doesn't matter when you take your vitamin supplement, but most of my patients seem to tolerate it better if they take it with their meal instead of with a supplement.

- One-A-Day Maximum Formula (my favorite)
- Centrum
- Spectrum Plus Minerals No Frills
- Theragran-M (low in calcium, but you get plenty of calcium in the weight-loss phase diet)

Fluids

It is *essential* that you drink at least 64 ounces of fluid each day. This fluid can be in the form of iced tea, diet sodas, diet fruit-flavored drinks (Crystal Light, Sugar-Free Kool Aid, and others), mineral water, coffee, and plain water—never fruit juices or nondiet sodas. These drinks are virtually all water with in some cases very small amounts of added flavoring and/or carbonation. You will be consuming large amounts of protein, the breakdown products of which must be excreted in the urine. Also, the fat that your body will be breaking down to meet your energy needs produces substances that must be gotten rid of in the urine. For these reasons, it is absolutely necessary for you to drink at least two quarts of fluid daily. You must provide your body with the fluids necessary to produce sufficient urine to remove these waste products. The fluids that you use to prepare your supplements are included in this 64 ounces.

Many patients tell me as I go over this with them, "Don't worry, I'm always drinking iced tea (or diet drinks, water, or whatever) throughout the day, so I'll get plenty of fluids." I always worry. I found from my own experience and from that of many patients that for some reason many people on the PSMF are not as thirsty as they normally are, and that they often don't take in the required amount of fluid. *Don't assume that you're taking in 64 ounces daily. Make sure.* You don't have to make elaborate calculations, but each afternoon think about how much fluid you've consumed to that point, and if it is under 32 ounces, make up for it during the remainder of the day.

Exercise

There is an entire chapter, Chapter 13, devoted to the function of exercise in weight loss, so I'm not going to go into great detail on the subject here. It is important that you read Chapter 13, especially the part dealing with pulse-driven exercise, and try to walk or do some other continuous exercise for at least 30 minutes, five days per week. This is not so much to aid in weight loss as it is to keep your metabolic rate from decreasing while you're on the PSMF.

Dining Out, Business, and Traveling
While on the PSMF

Many people on the PSMF will want to continue with a social life that often involves eating in restaurants, many need to pursue businesses that require lunches with customers and other kinds of entertaining, and many are in positions that require daily travel. The weight-loss phase diet is well suited to all these situations.

Most restaurants serve steak and salad, which are suitable for the meal. Often they will allow you to substitute broccoli or another allowable vegetable for the baked potato, but you must forsake the bread. You may have a mineral water such as Perrier with a twist of lemon instead of an alcoholic beverage, and even *occasionally* a small glass of champagne or dry white wine. Most friends, clients, or customers will never know you're dieting.

If you are on the road, it's no problem to take a shaker jar, buy diet drinks, and prepare your supplement along the way. Sometimes, however, in out-of-the-way places it is difficult to find steaks or seafood prepared in a suitable manner. On these occasions it is permissible to frequent one of the many fast-food outlets that are found everywhere. You may have a hamburger steak with a salad, or fried chicken with the skin removed, or even a double hamburger with mustard—jettison the bun. Keep in mind that you're not going to lose weight as quickly if you eat like this regularly because fried foods—no matter how carefully you try to de-skin or de-fat them —have many more calories than those prepared by baking, broiling, or grilling.

There are a few things you can do to make it easier on yourself when dining out. First, ask the waiter not to bring bread, potatoes, or rice—if you have that option. If not, and they come, take them and throw them away if you can discreetly or at least cover them with your napkin. If you sit and talk or have coffee after the meal, you will pick at the bread if it is sitting in front of you. Why not avoid the temptation? Second, try not to order anything that comes with potato chips, crackers, or other munchies because it is difficult not to nibble on them, and they are crawling with both fat and carbohydrates. Finally, don't even go near the dessert cart.

Monitoring Your Progress on the PSMF

In planning anything—whether it be a new business, a new marketing campaign, a plan to organize your life, a weight-loss plan, or even a plan to drive home from the grocery store—there are certain steps you must take to insure your success in the venture. You must first identify your starting position, and second, identify your goal. You then prepare a plan of action that will take you from your starting place to your goal within a *realistic* period of time. Finally, you must put in place some kind of periodic monitoring procedure that will inform you of your incremental progress toward your goal so that you can make minor modifications in your plan as you go along to insure your success. You should follow this outline for success during the weight-loss or PSMF phase of this program.

You know your starting weight, and from Chapter 4, your percent body fat; you also know, again from Chapter 4, your ideal body-fat range as a function of your age, and the weight in pounds that represents this ideal body-fat percentage. You have a plan— the PSMF—that if followed will take you from where you are now to where you want to be. Now, let's look at some ways that you can monitor your progress, and some modifications you can make as you go along to keep you moving toward your goal.

The easiest, most obvious way to keep track of your progress is by watching your weight on the scales. As long as you are losing on schedule—2 to 5 pounds per week—you don't need to worry, because, if you are adhering to the PSMF as instructed, you will be losing primarily body fat. If you are nibbling, drinking alcoholic beverages, adding extra carbohydrate to your diet, or otherwise not adhering to the regimen, all bets are off. You must stick *exactly* to the PSMF program and still not lose before you think about any modification.

This whole business of cheating can drive a doctor crazy. I have taken care of thousands of patients on this program—more than enough to make me aware of what typically happens. Almost all patients do well, but occasionally some come in mildly apprehensive, fearing that they haven't lost, and after weighing and finding that they are lighter, they exclaim, "I can't believe I lost this week because I really cheated." Or they may come in and state boldly at the outset, "I cheated all week, so I know I haven't lost." These patients don't cause me concern, because they know exactly what they did wrong, and how to correct the problem. They are accepting the blame for their failure to stick with their plan—the only modification they need make is to start doing the regimen correctly.

The patients who cause the grief are the ones who come in and haven't lost—or who may have even gained—and steadfastly insist that they haven't deviated from the plan by one iota. I'm not talking about a one-week setback, I'm talking about patients who come in week after week and don't lose. And based upon my experience with an enormous number of patients on the PSMF, I can categorically state that if a person rigidly adheres to the regimen, he or she will lose weight. If they don't lose, they aren't following the plan. These patients who come in repeatedly, complaining that the PSMF isn't working for them, are either trying to fool me or are fooling themselves. I counsel them, and most ultimately admit that they are indeed cheating and take the responsibility for their failure to do well, but some refuse to admit any deviation and try to shift the blame for their not doing well to me or to the PSMF. As I write this, one particular patient comes to mind, and although her story has a happy ending—thanks to fate, I suppose—most that involve similar patients don't.

Jean P., a forty-nine-year-old lady who was substantially overweight, started the PSMF and did well—the first week. After that, she either lost under a pound a week or sometimes didn't lose at all. She made several appointments to see me about her failure to lose and broke them all. Once she appeared without an appointment when I wasn't in the office and became loud and angry with my receptionist. Upon being informed of this, I set up a meeting with Ms. P. to discuss her problems with the diet.

We finally got together after several more broken appointments and had what could be called at the very least a memorable session. Ms. P. condemned the PSMF, my running of the clinic, and my abilities as a physician. Once she had vented her spleen—and likely the eardrums of everyone within a hundred-foot radius—we began to discuss her problems with the program. She insisted that she had been following it to the letter, and at that point, I wasn't about to contradict her. I made some minor modifications in her regimen and begged her not to vary from the program in the least.

"Doctor, I always do *exactly* as you instruct, and I will continue to do so, but we had better see results."

"I know you do, Ms. P.," I said, "and if you stick to this new, modified plan and don't lose anything this next week, maybe this isn't the diet plan for you. Come back and see me in a week, and if you haven't made progress, we'll look at some other options. But please, stick exactly with—"

"Doctor, I haven't cheated yet," she cut me off, "and I don't plan to start this week."

Seldom do things ever work out in real life as satisfactorily as the Ms. P. problem did. The day after this huge confrontation, my wife and I happened to be in a McDonald's having coffee when Ms. P. came through the door and walked to the counter. She ordered the largest ice cream cone available, then started eating it even before she had received her change. As she headed to the door, she saw me watching her, looked startled, and walked out. It was an embarrassing moment for both of us, but I will admit to having felt a little triumphant.

I fully expected never to see Ms. P. in the office again, but she was there the very next day. She apologized profusely for her behavior during her previous appointment, and she readily admitted that she had continuously cheated since the first week of her diet. I hope that if I am ever on the other side of an incident similar to this one, I handle myself with as much dignity and presence as did Ms. P. She resumed her program, picked up where she had left off after the first week, and lost to her goal weight. She maintained her weight for at least four months, after which she moved to another state, and we lost contact.

The point of this story is that you shouldn't accuse the plan of not working if you're not following it. Don't try to make modifications in the regimen if what is needed is a modification in your behavior. All the monitoring and modifications I will discuss from this point on will assume that you are following the regimen exactly as outlined.

If you are losing at least two pounds or more a week, *on the average*, keep doing what you're doing. Try to weigh early in the morning after you have emptied your bladder, and before you get dressed. Weigh once a week, not every day. After you have lost half the weight that you calculated that you needed to lose, recalculate your percent bodyfat, your lean-body mass, and your goal weight. You may find that your goal weight has changed. You may have gained some lean body mass if you have started an exercise program, or you may find that you have lost some lean body mass if your overall weight loss has been large—in either case your goal weight must be readjusted.

Even though you may be weighing every week and doing well, I urge you to check your progress also by trying on clothing that is too small as discussed at the end of Chapter 4. As long as you continue to be able to wear smaller and smaller clothing, you are doing well regardless of what the scales show. You should only think about modifying the regimen if (1) you are not losing scale weight, *and* (2) your clothing is not fitting more loosely (since clothing fit can be a subjective thing, I would check hip and waist measurement changes before declaring with certainty that I was not getting smaller). Don't throw up your hands and decide to change if you have a bad week, because that's going to happen—modify the regimen only after several weeks without much change.

In my clinic, I determine the degree to which I modify the regimen by routinely checking the level of ketosis of all my patients weekly. You can do this yourself at home and use the results to gauge your progress.

Ketosis and the PSMF

One of the main reasons the PSMF is so successful is that people can stay on it for long periods of time without being hungry. The thought that probably crossed your mind the first time you heard about someone's being on the PSMF was how they could consume a small meal and a few shakes every day—and nothing else—and not be ravenously hungry. The reason for this lack of hunger is that people on the PSMF are typically in ketosis. We touched on ketosis briefly in Chapter 2, but now let's discuss it in a little more detail and learn its role in the PSMF regimen.

What exactly are ketones, and what does it mean to be in ketosis? When your body breaks down its fat stores for energy *in the absence of carbohydrates,* ketones, or ketoacids, are formed. This happens because of the way our bodies are put together biochemically. We have many different biochemical systems to deal with the breakdown and transformation of various biological materials. We can look at some of these pathways as machines that use different substances for fuel and produce energy and fuel-breakdown products. The machine or pathway our body uses depends upon which fuel is available. If both carbohydrates and fat are available in the diet, one pathway is used; if no carbohydrate is available, another is used. The pathway that is used by the body to break down body fat with little or no dietary carbohydrate produces, among other things, ketones as a by-product. The ketones that are produced are small molecules with an acidic configuration, and these are more correctly called ketoacids. They can be used by the brain, and to an extent, the other tissues, for fuel after a period of adaptation. Mainly, however, they are eliminated in the urine, in the breath, and in the stool. Ketones, in most cases, exert an effect on our mood and make us experience a degree of euphoria, while at the same time preventing us from being hungry.

This hunger-slacking, or "anorectic," to use the medical term, property of ketones is what allows us to follow the PSMF for long periods of time without being especially hungry. Even though ketosis (the state of having ketones circulating in the blood) theoretically protects against hunger, I would not be telling you the truth if I said that as soon as you get in ketosis, you will never be hungry again. You will occasionally be hungry, but you should almost never have that ravenous hunger that we're all so familiar with while dieting. Most of the time you shouldn't be hungry at all, the rest of the time your hunger should be manageable. If you are hungry all the time, or if you are failing to lose weight and size as discussed above, then you need to check your level of ketosis.

Checking for Ketones

Of the three places ketones can be found—the breath, urine, and stool—the urine is the easiest to check. First, you must purchase a bottle of Ketostix or something comparable. Tell your pharmacist that you want to test for ketones in your urine, and he or she can provide you with the proper test strips. Ketostix are small, plastic test strips—about three inches long, and one-fourth of an inch wide—that have a small pad of chemically impregnated substance on the end. This pad is a very light, almost yellowish, tan color, and when exposed to ketones, it turns purple. The degree of ketosis is indicated by the intensity of the purple—the deeper and darker the purple, the heavier the ketosis.

Once you have the Ketostix, you can monitor your level of ketosis regularly. Catch a sample of your urine in a small cup and then dip the test strip into it. Remove the strip and wait several seconds—if the strip turns purple to any extent at all, you're in ketosis. Your level of ketosis can vary throughout the day and can be influenced by any carbohydrates you consume, so if you are not in ketosis when you first check, try again later in the day.

As long as you are losing weight and are not incredibly hungry all the time, there is no real reason to make checking your ketones a ritual. You may, just out of interest, want to check them, but there is no compelling reason to do so. You will, however, need to check for ketones when you make the transition onto the maintenance diet. If things are going great for you and you check your level of ketosis and find it nonexistent—what then? Leave things alone, don't try to modify anything—if it's not broken, don't try to fix it. But if things aren't going great, and you're not in ketosis, you may need to modify the regimen slightly.

Modifying the Weight-Loss Regimen

If you aren't losing well, or if you are hungry all the time, or worst of all, if you're both not losing *and* you're hungry constantly, you might need to change your supplement. But first, make sure you are getting no extra carbohydrate from any other source. For example, I have had patients who were drinking orange juice—26 grams of carbohydrate per glass—or were, incredible as it sounds, mixing their supplements in nondiet soft drinks. Before you change the supplement, review your diet and be certain that you are consuming no carbohydrates other than those in the supplements or the tiny amount in the meal. If this is the case and you are not doing well on the PSMF—and this will be a *very* few people—you need to modify the basic supplement slightly by decreasing the amount of carbohydrate.

The supplement as described contains 48 grams of carbohydrate in the powdered milk, 3 grams in the fructose, and anywhere from 0 to 6 or 8 grams in the protein powder, depending upon the powder you're using—providing a total of from 51 grams to 59 grams per day. The first way in which you should try to decrease the carbohydrates is by converting to a protein powder containing no carbohydrates. If this doesn't work, or if you are already using a no-carbohydrate protein powder, you may start slightly reducing the amount of powdered milk. You may, in increments, reduce the powdered milk until you either go into ketosis or start losing weight and feeling less hungry. Don't decrease the powdered milk to less than one-half the starting amount. At one-half the starting amount, you have reduced the carbohydrate content of the day's supplements by 24 grams. If you are still having trouble, discuss the problem with your physician.

Questions About the PSMF

Since the PSMF is very different from any diet you have ever encountered, you may have several questions at this point. Since I have presented this diet to several thousand patients, I have become familiar with the questions and concerns most people have. I will try to answer most of these in a question-and-answer format.

Q. May I have the meal divided into two portions instead of eating it all at once?
A. Yes, just make sure that you don't eat more than what is allowed by dividing your meal.

Q. Do I have to take all the supplements?
A. Yes. It is essential that you get the necessary protein and other nutrients that are a part of the supplements. If you don't, then you risk the problems that people had while on a total fast or on the liquid protein as described in Chapter 2.

Q. What if I can't get all four supplements down in a day?

A. This, surprisingly enough, is a problem that many encounter. People on the PSMF are often so unhungry that they forget to eat. Before they know it, it is late in the afternoon and they have had only one supplement, and that in the morning. They consume another supplement and then eat their meal shortly after. They are then confronted with having to drink two supplements before bedtime. Most just drink one and promise to do better the next day. If this happens to you a time or two, or if you even have only two supplements in a day once in a while, it's no big deal. The problem comes when people chronically consume only two or three. If you find this happening to you, double up on your supplements—mix two with your diet beverage, and this should solve your problem.

Q. What if I can't stand the taste of the supplements?

A. The component of the supplement mixture that causes the taste problem for almost all the people who have a problem is the protein portion. If you try a protein powder and don't like the supplement it makes—switch protein powders. There are a multitude on the market with a wide variation in taste, so keep trying until you find one that you can tolerate. I can tell you from experience that there is no single one that is universally loved or hated. There is a tremendous variation in people's tastes where protein powder is concerned.

Q. I am on blood-pressure medicines, what should I do?

A. You should discuss your medications with your doctor. As you will see in Chapter 11, the PSMF generally decreases elevated blood pressure, and depending upon the underlying cause of your high blood pressure, your physician may start reducing your medicine as you proceed on the diet. DON'T TRY TO ADJUST YOUR MEDICINE WITHOUT YOUR PHYSICIAN'S KNOWLEDGE AND RECOMMENDATION!

Q. What if I am taking medicine for diabetes?

A. This regimen works well for type II diabetics who are on oral medications, but once again—DON'T TRY TO CHANGE YOUR MEDICINES WITHOUT YOUR PHYSICIAN'S KNOWLEDGE. If your physician isn't comfortable taking care of you while you are on the PSMF, ask him or her to refer you to a physician who is, or see Appendix A to find a physician yourself.

Q. May I go on the PSMF if I have high cholesterol?

A. Yes. Most of the time cholesterol is reduced dramatically on this regimen and on the low-carbohydrate maintenance plan. Chapter 11 will provide more specifics on the cholesterol issue.

Q. What can I do if I get in a situation where I have no supplements available?

A. This can happen occasionally. If it does, eat two to three ounces of meat of your choice and a small salad in place of the missing supplement. For breakfast, you may substitute two boiled eggs for the meat and do without the salad. You should stay in ketosis on this regimen and continue to feel fine, but get back to the supplements as soon as you can to get the calcium and other nutrients.

Q. I've heard that ketosis causes bad breath and sometimes headaches, is that true?

A. Yes, it is true. You can chew sugarless gum or use breath spray to overcome the bad breath. Usually a couple of Tylenol tablets will get rid of the headache, but you need to discuss it with your physician if it persists. Earlier when we discussed ketones, we dealt mainly with the situation in which someone was unable to get into ketosis. Some people have the opposite problem and get into heavy ketosis, which can sometimes cause headaches and/or sleeplessness. If you are having problems with headaches or sleeplessness and you check and find your ketone level to be very high, you can add some more fructose to your supplements and try to moderate your level of ketosis. There is a wide variation among people in their sensitivity to carbohydrates as far as going into ketosis is concerned. Some people are very sensitive and even 30 grams will keep them out, but others can tolerate 90 to 100 grams and still be in ketosis. You may have to adjust your supplement accordingly, but only if you're having a problem.

Q. What other problems or side effects might I have on the PSMF?

A. Most people sail through the PSMF without having any significant problems, but occasionally minor problems such as constipation, dizziness, irritability, and others may occur. I have included an entire chapter—Chapter 12—on these minor problems and how to deal with them. Chapter 12 includes the same information that I give patients in my clinic when they start the PSMF. As I do them, I encourage you to read the information in Chapter 12 before you begin the PSMF.

7

In Transition

*B*Y now, you should be close to your goal weight, and your body fat percentage should be in or near the ideal range for your age. It is time for you to begin weaning from the PSMF and make your transition into the maintenance phase, which you should follow for the rest of your life. You accomplish this weaning by shifting from a PSMF composed of supplements and a meal to a PSMF-like diet made entirely of food. To this diet, which is high in protein but very low in carbohydrate, you will start to add carbohydrate gradually until you have reached your maintenance level. Along the way, you should lose the remainder of any excess fat you still carry and reach your goal weight. This chapter will instruct you specifically in how to make this transition from the PSMF to your maintenance diet.

You may be hesitant to stop the PSMF, because, if you are like most of my patients, you will be feeling better than you have in a long time, and you will be accustomed to never having to think about what you're going to eat for most of your meals. You may also experience some anxiety at this point because you fear that if you start eating again, you will proceed to regain all your lost weight. I can assure you that if you follow the instructions in this chapter, you will not regain your weight. Granted, you will have to expend a little more effort on food preparation during the transitional and maintenance phases than you did on the PSMF, but at some point you are going to have to resume eating, and it's no more trouble to prepare these menus than any others.

Because it has been so simple to follow, many patients ask me if they can stay on the PSMF forever. Even though the supplements, with meal and multivitamin supplementation, are a complete food, I discourage the use of the PSMF beyond the weight-loss phase. Unlike our Paleolithic ancestors, who ate mainly for survival (although I'm sure they enjoyed it), we eat primarily for pleasure, and since most of us have ready access to easily obtainable foods, only secondarily for survival. The enjoyment of food is one of life's great pleasures, so why deny it to ourselves? The reason is that most people equate the consumption of delicious food with gaining weight, and in many cases they are correct, but it doesn't have to be that way. The maintenance diet, and to a certain extent the transitional diet, provide large quantities of rich, flavorful, and nutritious food for us to savor, but at the same time they allow us to maintain our goal weight (which is now our normal weight). Look upon the PSMF, simple and effective though it was, as a milestone passed, and let's move on toward maintenance.

Basic Transitional Diet

To begin the transitional phase, you must limit your intake of carbohydrates to 20 grams a day. Even with this restriction, you can still enjoy a delicious diet with a fair amount of variety. You must stick to the transitional diet closely and hold off on the promised dietary vacations until you reach maintenance. The purpose of the transitional phase is to take you from a low-calorie/low-carbohydrate diet designed to help you lose weight (the PSMF) to a higher-calorie/low-carbohydrate diet designed to help you maintain your weight. You will accomplish this transition by restricting your carbohydrate intake to an even lower level than on the PSMF while at the same time increasing your caloric intake. You will then gradually increase your carbohydrate intake in 20-gram increments until you reach your maintenance level. In this chapter, I give you a basic diet framework and instructions to use to build your own menus—tailored to your particular tastes. Some of you—like many of my patients—may prefer to follow exact menus that guide you through the various levels of carbohydrate intake. For you, I have prepared a full week of meal plans at the 20-gram level, the 40-gram level, and the 60-gram level. These can be found at the end of this chapter, beginning on page 123.

THE BASIC TRANSITION (AND RECOVERY) DIET

Breakfast
2 eggs, any style
8 oz Sugar-Free Tang
coffee or tea

Lunch
1 cup salad
4–6 oz lean meat
or
Tuna or Chicken Salad*
iced tea, or diet beverage

Supper
2 cups salad
or 1 cup broccoli
8 oz meat, fish, or fowl
coffee, tea, or diet beverage

To this basic nearly zero-carbohydrate framework, you should add 4–6 ounces of any kind of hard cheese (cheddar, Swiss, Muenster, Colby, Havarti, etc.) and 2 slices of low-carbohydrate bread (such as Colonial Light brand white or wheat, which has only 6 grams per slice). You may add them at any point along the day that suits you: for example, the bread slices can be toasted and eaten with butter at breakfast, or, if you prefer, used to make a sandwich with the tuna salad, chicken salad, or the meat and eaten for lunch. These additional items bring the total daily carbohydrate intake to approximately 20 grams, which is the level at which you will begin the transition to maintenance.

It is essential that you eat the 4–6 ounces of cheese daily as

*see recipe section of Chapter 9

outlined because it provides a large portion of your daily calcium requirement. While you are on the transition diet, especially during the early stages, you will still be producing ketones. These ketones are acids and consequently cause your blood to be slightly acidic. Acid in the blood is buffered by, among other things, calcium ions, which come from your main calcium storehouse—your bones. This calcium, along with the ketones, is eliminated via the urine. While on a diet, such as this one, that results in your being in ketosis, you must take in additional calcium in your diet in order to maintain total body calcium equilibrium. Because of this propensity to lose calcium, if you have an allergy to dairy products and can't eat the cheese, you should take a calcium supplement during this phase of the diet.

Many patients ask me about coffee, tea, and diet beverages. I don't see any problem in your consuming these products in whatever quantities you want, within reason. I don't think that it's necessary to have decaffeinated coffee, tea, or diet drinks as long as you don't have a problem with caffeine. If you have stomach problems that coffee makes worse, don't drink it. Otherwise, I don't think you need to limit yourself to only one cup in the morning, or any other time—just use good judgment.

You will remain at this 20-gram carbohydrate level for two weeks. As we will discuss in great detail in the next chapter, you will also return to this level for a day or two to "recover" from any later bouts of dietary indiscretion to which you may fall victim.

During the transition diet you may use butter, mayonnaise, sugar-free sweeteners, and any other foods that contain no carbohydrates pretty much as you see fit. Continue to restrict your use of alcohol, however, until you complete your transition to your maintenance level. Although according to the carbohydrate-counting books, alcohol contains no carbohydrate, it does exert a "carbohydratelike" effect, so limit its use.

After the first two weeks of transition, you will increase your daily intake of carbohydrate from 20 grams to 40 grams. To be able to do this, you must have a book listing the carbohydrate content of various foods. Several are listed in Appendix B. Don't worry at this point about the Effective Carbohydrate Content (you will learn about this in Chapter 8) of the foods; just use the carbohydrate figures as listed in the books you purchase. Your mission here is to add an additional 15–20 grams of carbohydrate to your daily dietary intake. The choice of foods is entirely yours. If you have been craving a particular food, search it out in the book and treat yourself to a 20-gram serving of it. Enjoy yourself, you've earned the pleasure! Remain at a daily intake of 40 grams for one week.

In the fifth and sixth weeks—your last weeks of transition—you will again increase your daily intake of carbohydrates another 20 grams. Just as you did before, find another item or combination of items totaling 20 grams in carbohydrate content and add this to last week's diet. Your daily intake of carbohydrate is now 60 grams. Remain at this level for two weeks.

During the last three days of this sixth week of transition, you will want to check your urine for ketones at several intervals during the day. If you can no longer detect ketones in your urine at any time during the day on a 60-gram daily intake of carbohydrates, then go no further and remain at approximately 60 grams as your maintenance level on a daily basis. If, however, you still find ketones in your urine, you can tolerate a higher daily intake of carbohydrates. Continue weekly to add carbohydrate in 15–20 gram increments until you can no longer detect ketones in your urine. Most individuals tolerate between 60 and 90 grams per day.

The 60-gram (or higher if you are still in ketosis at 60 grams) daily carbohydrate diet puts you approximately where you need to be as far as carbohydrate intake is concerned, but only approximately. You need to fine-tune your diet until you find the carbohydrate intake that allows you to maintain your weight precisely where you want it, and this you will learn to do in the next chapter.

Before we forge ahead, however, let's look at some commonly asked questions about the transitional diet.

Q. Do I need to continue drinking all the fluids daily?

A. Yes. The transition diet is a high-protein diet and as such requires that enough urine be made to carry away the protein-breakdown products. You must continue to drink at least 64 ounces of fluids both on the transitional *and* on the maintenance diets.

Q. Should I continue to take my multivitamin tablet daily once I'm off the PSMF?

A. Continue to take your vitamin while on the transitional diet, but once on maintenance you will get enough food variety that you shouldn't need supplemental vitamins to prevent deficiency problems. Many people, however, continue to take a multivitamin while on maintenance, and I don't have any argument with that.

Q. How long can I stay on the PSMF?

A. I have had patients in my clinic who were extremely obese and who stayed on the PSMF for twelve to sixteen months without difficulty. I monitored these patients closely and was prepared to make changes in their regimen if a problem became evident. You should discuss your case with your physician as you progress, letting him or her make the decision as to how long you stay on the PSMF. The regimen as described in this book is modified in such a way as to enhance its safety, so I don't see a problem in your staying on the plan *exactly as instructed* until you reach your goal weight. Some recent evidence suggests that dieters who remain on the PSMF for extended periods (a year or more) become depleted of O-3 fatty acids. This should not happen to you if you occasionally eat cold-water fish such as salmon or mackerel as the meat portion of your meal. You may wish to take the BioSyn supplements described in Chapter 10 to avoid this deficiency problem and for the health benefits they provide.

Q. What if I'm allergic to cheese? How do I get my 4–6 ounces daily that I need for the calcium?

A. If you have a cheese allergy, you must take a calcium supplement. Ask your pharmacist for a brand that's available in your area that will give you at least 1,500 mgs per day of readily absorbable calcium.

Q. I'm not a big bread eater. Do I have to have the 2 slices of Colonial Light or Wonder Light bread daily?

A. You are very lucky that you don't particularly like bread—you should do well on a low-carbohydrate diet. If you don't want the bread, substitute for it any vegetable that has about 10 grams of carbohydrate per serving.

Q. What happens if I gain weight on the transition diet?

A. You shouldn't gain weight at all. In fact, you should continue to lose, although more slowly than you did on the PSMF. If you gain weight, make absolutely certain that you are following the transition diet to the letter. The few patients I have had that had this happen were all, without exception, not following the diet as outlined.

Congratulations, you are now ready to proceed to maintenance, where the real challenge begins.

Now, as promised, here are the specific menu plans for those of you who prefer them.

You should remain at each of the carbohydrate levels for two weeks—repeating days 1 through 7, or choosing your favorite days and repeating them. Please do repeat the entire day's menu, since the plans are designed to approximate the specified carbohydrate allotment for the day as a whole. If you should need to substitute a dish for whatever reason, make certain that the carbohydrate grams in the alternate dish are less than or equal to what it replaces—I have indicated at the right of the meal plans the carbohydrate content in grams for those dishes containing more than a negligible amount. Please note that many of the dishes are marked with an asterisk—this indicates that the recipe for this dish can be found in Chapter 9.

Sample Daily Menus
For the Transition Phase

Weeks 1 And 2—20-Gram Level

Day 1

CARBOHYDRATE
GRAMS

Breakfast
2 eggs, scrambled†
2 links sausage
6 oz Sugar-Free Tang
coffee or tea

Lunch
turkey breast sandwich
(made with 4 oz turkey breast meat,
2 slices Colonial or Wonder light wheat toast,   12
mustard, mayo, lettuce, tomato slices,
and 2 oz Swiss cheese)   2
iced tea or diet beverage

Snack
2 oz Swiss cheese   2
sugar-free beverage

†I recommend using canola oil for all frying.

Supper
2 cups mixed green salad
1 oz Italian Dressing*   1
Rosemary Chicken Breasts*   1
1 cup steamed broccoli or cauliflower   4
coffee, tea, or diet beverage

Day 2

Breakfast
3-egg cheese omelette
(made with 2 oz shredded cheddar cheese)   2
1 slice Colonial or Wonder light wheat toast and butter   6
6 oz Sugar-Free Tang
coffee or tea

Lunch
mixed salad
(made with lettuce, 3 oz beef or turkey,
and 2 oz Swiss cheese)   13
2 saltine crackers and butter   4
iced tea or diet beverage

Snack
4 oz Sugar-Free Jell-O gelatin
(optional)

Supper
French Onion Pork Chop*   4
1 cup mixed salad greens and allowable dressing
1 cup steamed broccoli   4
coffee, tea, or diet beverage

Day 3

Breakfast
2 scrambled eggs
2 strips lean bacon
6 oz Sugar-Free Tang or mineral water
coffee or tea

Lunch
Tuna Salad* Sandwich   14
(on 2 slices Colonial or Wonder light wheat bread
with mayo, mustard, lettuce, tomato if desired)
2 oz sliced Muenster cheese   2
1 cup chicken or beef bouillon
sugar-free beverage

Snack
2 oz Muenster cheese   2

Supper
1 serving Kaye's Quiche*   3
2 cups tossed green salad
1 oz low-carbohydrate dressing
sugar-free beverage or mineral water
coffee or tea

Day 4

Breakfast
2 poached eggs on buttered toast
(using 1 slice, halved, Colonial or Wonder light bread)   6
2 pieces lean bacon
6 oz Sugar-Free Tang or mineral water
coffee or tea

Lunch
1 serving Kaye's Quiche (left from dinner)   3
1 cup salad greens topped with
2 oz shredded Muenster cheese   2
1 oz low-carbohydrate dressing
sugar-free beverage or mineral water

Snack
1 cup beef bouillon
(optional)

Supper
1 serving Fish and Peppers*   2
1 cup steamed cauliflower   4
(topped with 2 oz melted shredded cheddar cheese)   2

Sugar-Free Jell-O gelatin
sugar-free beverage, coffee, or tea

Day 5

Breakfast
1 slice cheddar cheese toast   7
(made with 1-oz slice cheddar cheese
melted atop 1 slice buttered Colonial or Wonder light toast)
2 links sausage
6 oz Sugar-Free Tang or mineral water
coffee or tea

Lunch
1 serving Chicken Salad*   2
1 cup tossed salad
1 oz allowable dressing
3 saltine crackers   6
sugar-free beverage, coffee, or tea

Snack
2 oz Havarti cheese   2

Supper
1 serving French Onion Chicken Breasts*   2
½ cup steamed zucchini, buttered   3
4 oz Sugar-Free Jell-O gelatin
sugar-free beverage or mineral water
coffee or tea

Day 6

Breakfast
2-egg ham-and-cheese omelette
(made with 2 oz each diced ham and cheddar cheese)   2
1 slice Colonial or Wonder light toast and butter   6
6 oz Sugar-Free Tang or mineral water

Lunch
1 piece cold leftover French Onion Chicken   2
1 cup salad greens topped with

2 oz shredded Havarti cheese   2
1 oz allowable dressing
sugar-free beverage

Snack
1 cup chicken or beef bouillon
(optional)

Supper
1 serving Avgolemono Soup*   1
1 serving Cinder's Lemon Chicken*   6
1 cup steamed broccoli   4
sugar-free beverage, coffee, or tea

Day 7

Breakfast
2 scrambled eggs with butter
2 links sausage
6 oz Sugar-Free Tang or mineral water
coffee or tea

Lunch
grilled cheese sandwich
(made with 2 oz Havarti or cheddar cheese on   14
2 slices buttered Colonial or Wonder light wheat bread)
1 cup Avgolemono Soup (from yesterday)   1
sugar-free beverage, mineral water, or tea

Snack
4 oz Sugar-Free Jell-O gelatin
(optional)

Supper
1 serving Skillet Chicken Italiano*   7
½ cup steamed zucchini   3
1 cup salad greens
1 oz allowable salad dressing
sugar-free beverage, mineral water, or tea
coffee

Weeks 3 and 4—40-Gram Level

Day 1

Breakfast
3-egg bacon-and-cheese omelette
(made with 2 slices bacon and 2 oz Swiss cheese) 2
1 slice buttered Colonial or Wonder light toast 6
6 oz Sugar-Free Tang or mineral water
coffee or tea

Lunch
Chef's Salad (see page 134) 12
2 oz allowable salad dressing 2
sugar-free beverage, mineral water, or tea

Snack
½ cup plain yogurt 7
(sweetened with 1 packet Equal sweetener)

Supper
1 serving Mom's Meat Loaf* 8
1 serving Sautéed Broccoli* 4
2 deviled-egg halves
sugar-free beverage, mineral water, or tea
coffee

Day 2

Breakfast
2 poached eggs on toast
(on 1 slice, halved, Colonial or Wonder light toast) 6
2 links sausage
6 oz Sugar-Free Tang or mineral water
coffee or tea

Lunch
Mom's Meat Loaf Sandwich 4
(made with 1"-slice meat loaf and 2 slices 12
Colonial or Wonder light bread)
mayo, mustard, dill pickle (optional)

2 deviled-egg halves
sugar-free beverage, mineral water, tea

Snack
2 oz cheddar cheese   2

Supper
1 serving Sunday Spicy Chicken*   2
1 serving Herbed Brussels Sprouts*   8
½ tomato, sliced and topped with Italian Dressing   4
(and topped with 1 oz grated parmesan cheese)   1
sugar-free beverage, mineral water, or tea
coffee

Day 3

Breakfast
1 serving Quaker Instant Oatmeal   18
topped with butter and Equal sweetener
and ¼ cup warm milk   3
6 oz Sugar-Free Tang or mineral water
coffee or tea

Lunch
Tuna Salad   2
2 oz Havarti cheese   2
1 cup tossed salad
1 oz allowable dressing
4 saltine crackers   8
sugar-free beverage, mineral water, or tea

Snack
1 cup beef bouillon
(optional)

Supper
1 serving Chicken Tabasco*   1
1 cup chopped broccoli topped with   5
butter and 1 oz grated parmesan cheese
4 oz Sugar-Free Jell-O gelatin
sugar-free beverage, mineral water, or tea
coffee

Day 4

Breakfast
2 eggs, scrambled with 1 oz diced ham
1 slice cheddar cheese toast   7
(made with Colonial or Wonder light bread topped with
1 oz cheddar cheese, melted)
6 oz Sugar-Free Tang or mineral water
coffee or tea

Lunch
1 piece leftover cold Chicken Tabasco (last night's)   1
1 cup mixed green salad topped with
2 oz shredded Muenster cheese and 1 slice crumbled bacon 2
1 oz allowable salad dressing
sugar-free beverage, mineral water, or tea

Snack
½ cup plain yogurt   7
(sweetened with 1 packet Equal sweetener)

Supper
1 serving Easy Pork Tenderloin*   2
½ apple, cooked   9
(cook in pat butter, sprinkle with Equal and a dash cinnamon)
1 serving Seasoned Green Beans*   5
sugar-free beverage, mineral water, or tea

Dessert
4 oz sugar-free French vanilla pudding   8
coffee

Day 5

Breakfast
2 slices Almost Cinnamon Toast   12
(sprinkle ½ tsp cinnamon and 1/2 packet Equal
onto 2 slices Colonial or Wonder light bread
already toasted and buttered)
2 links sausage
6 oz whole fresh milk   8
coffee or tea

Lunch
2 cups salad greens topped with 1 chopped hard-boiled egg,
2 oz Swiss cheese and 2 oz leftover tenderloin   2
2 oz allowable dressing
½ cup Avgolemono Soup*   1
sugar-free beverage, mineral water, tea

Snack
1 oz Swiss cheese

Supper
1 serving Roast Pork Stir-fry*   12
1 cup steamed broccoli spears   4
sugar-free beverage or mineral water
hot tea

Dessert (optional)
4 oz Sugar-Free Jell-O gelatin
(topped with a dollop of whipped cream   1
sweetened with Equal or Sweet'N Low)
coffee

Day 6

Breakfast
2 Cracker Eggs
(made by crumbling 5 saltine crackers into a bowl,   10
topping with the poached eggs, and chopping
with a spoon to combine them)
2 pieces lean bacon
6 oz Sugar-Free Tang or mineral water
coffee or tea

Lunch
ham-and-cheese sandwich   13
(on two slices Colonial or Wonder light wheat bread,
made with 2 oz sliced ham, 1 oz sliced Swiss,
lettuce, tomato, mayo, mustard—as desired)
1 cup beef bouillon
sugar-free beverage, mineral water, or tea
coffee

Snack
½ cup plain yogurt   7
(sweetened with Equal or Sweet'N Low)

Supper
1 serving Weight-Loss Chili*   6
2 cups tossed green salad
1 oz allowable salad dressing
1 slice garlic cheese toast   7
(made by broiling 1 slice Colonial or Wonder light bread
spread with butter, sprinkled with garlic powder,
and topped with a sprinkle of parmesan cheese)
sugar-free beverage, mineral water, or tea
coffee

Day 7

Breakfast
2 poached eggs on buttered toast
(using 1 slice, halved, Colonial or Wonder light bread) 6
2 slices lean bacon
6 oz Sugar-Free Tang or mineral water
coffee or tea

Lunch
bacon, lettuce, and tomato sandwich
(on 2 slices Colonial or Wonder light toast   12
with 3 slices lean bacon, 1 oz Muenster cheese, tomato,
lettuce, mayo, mustard—as desired)
1 hard-boiled egg
2 dill pickle spears
4 oz sugar-free Jell-O gelatin
sugar-free beverage, mineral water, or tea

Snack (optional)
1 cup chicken bouillon
sugar-free beverage

Supper
1 serving Roman Style Chicken*   8
1 cup steamed broccoli   4

1 cup tossed green salad
1 oz allowable salad dressing
sugar-free beverage, mineral water, tea

Dessert (optional)

1 serving Strawberry Cheesecake*   4
coffee

• **Weeks 5 and 6—60-Gram Level**

Day 1

Breakfast

3-egg three-cheese omelette   3
(made with 1 oz each shredded cheddar, Swiss, Muenster)
2 or 3 sausage links
2 slices buttered Colonial or Wonder light wheat toast   12
6 oz. Sugar-Free Tang or mineral water
coffee or tea

Lunch

1 serving Homestyle Tomato Soup*   9
Tuna Salad* Sandwich   12
(made with 2 slices Colonial or Wonder light wheat bread)
sugar-free beverage, mineral water, or tea

Snack

½ crisp apple   11
1 oz cheddar cheese   1

Supper

1 serving Roasted Paprika Chicken*   4
1 cup Sautéed Broccoli*
1 cup tossed salad
1 oz allowable dressing
sugar-free beverage, mineral water, or tea

Dessert (optional)

1 serving Strawberry Cheesecake   4
coffee

Day 2

Breakfast
1 packet Quaker Instant Oatmeal   18
(sweetened with 1 packet Equal or Sweet'N Low
and topped with a sprinkle cinnamon
and ¼ cup warm milk)   3
2 strips lean bacon
6 oz Sugar-Free Tang or mineral water
coffee or tea

Lunch
Chef's Salad   12
(made with diced 2 oz Roasted Paprika Chicken
from last night and 1 oz diced Havarti or Swiss cheese and
1 sliced hard-boiled egg)
3 saltine crackers   6
2 oz allowable salad dressing
sugar-free beverage, mineral water, or tea

Snack
½ cup plain yogurt   7
topped with 2 tbsp Strawberry Preserves*   2
(sweeten with 1 packet Equal or Sweet'N Low if desired)

Supper
1 serving Shrimp Scampi*   2
1 serving Wilted Leaf Lettuce Salad*   3
1 slice garlic cheese toast   7
(broil 1 slice Colonial or Wonder light bread,
spread with butter, sprinkle with garlic powder,
and dust with parmesan cheese)
sugar-free beverage, mineral water, or tea

Dessert (optional)
4 oz. Sugar-Free Jell-O gelatin
topped with a dollop of whipped cream   1
(sweetened with Equal or Sweet'N Low)
coffee

Day 3

Breakfast
2 slices cheese toast   14
(made as previously directed)
2 links sausage
6 oz Sugar-Free Tang or mineral water

Lunch
Egg Salad* Sandwich
(made on 2 slices Colonial or Wonder light wheat bread)   12
2 dill pickle spears
1 serving Homestyle Tomato Soup*   9
sugar-free beverage, mineral water, or tea

Snack
2 oz cheddar cheese   2
sugar-free beverage

Supper
1 serving Hobo Dinner Pork Chops*   18
1 cup tossed salad
1 oz allowable salad dressing
sugar-free beverage, mineral water, or tea
coffee

Dessert (optional)
1 serving Hot Chocolate*   3

Day 4

Breakfast
2 poached eggs on buttered toast
(use 1 slice, halved, Colonial or Wonder light bread)   6
2 slices lean bacon
bananas and milk   19
(½ banana sliced, ½ cup whole milk
sweetened with 1 packet Equal or Sweet'N Low—if desired)

Lunch
Egg Salad Stuffed Tomato   7
(cut tomato almost through into six sections,

spread them apart, and fill with ½ cup Egg Salad, left from
yesterday)
1 oz allowable dressing—if desired
2 slices dill pickle
4 saltine crackers   8
sugar-free beverage, mineral water, or tea

Snack
1 cup chicken bouillon
(optional)

Supper
1 serving Rosemary Chicken*   2
1 serving Eggplant Milano*   6
1 cup steamed broccoli   4
(topped with 2 oz Italian Dressing vinaigrette if desired)
sugar-free beverage, mineral water, or tea

Dessert (optional)
2 squares Sinfully Rich Fudge*   4
coffee

Day 5

Breakfast
bananas and milk   19
(½ banana sliced, 1/2 cup whole milk
sweetened with 1 packet Equal or Sweet'N Low—if desired)
3 sausage links
6 oz Sugar-Free Tang or mineral water
coffee or tea

Lunch
Chicken Salad* Sandwich   14
(on 2 slices Colonial or Wonder light wheat bread
with lettuce, tomato, mayo, and mustard—if desired)
1 oz Havarti cheese   1
2 dill pickle spears
1 cup chicken bouillon
sugar-free beverage, mineral water, tea

Snack
2 oz Havarti cheese   2
sugar-free beverage

Supper
1 serving Mom's Meat Loaf*   8
1 serving Butter Lettuce Salad*   6
(or 1 cup tossed salad, optional)
1 serving Seasoned Green Beans*   5
sugar-free beverage, mineral water, or tea

Dessert (optional)
4 squares Sinfully Rich Fudge*   4
coffee

Day 6

Breakfast
2 slices Almost Cinnamon Toast   12
(sprinkle ½ tsp cinnamon and ½ packet Equal onto 2
slices Colonial or Wonder light bread
already toasted and buttered)
2 pieces lean bacon
6 oz Sugar-Free Tang or mineral water
coffee or tea

Lunch
Mom's Meat Loaf Sandwich (left over from supper)   4
(made on 2 slices Colonial or Wonder light bread   12
with lettuce, tomato, onion, mayo, and mustard—as desired)
1 hard-boiled egg
2 dill pickle spears
sugar-free beverage, mineral water, or tea

Snack
2 oz Swiss, cheddar, or Muenster cheese   2
½ crisp apple   11
Sugar-free beverage

Supper
1 serving French Onion Pork Chops*   4
½ apple, sauteed in butter and   11

sprinkled with ¼ tsp cinnamon and 1 packet Equal
1 serving Seasoned Green Beans (from yesterday)   5
1 cup tossed salad with allowable dressing (if desired)
sugar-free beverage, mineral water, or tea

Dessert (optional)
4 oz Sugar-Free Jell-O gelatin
topped with a dollop of whipped cream   1
(sweetened with Equal or Sweet'N Low)
coffee

Day 7

Breakfast
3-egg ham-and-cheese omelette   1
(made with 1 oz each diced ham and Swiss or cheddar)
2 slices buttered Colonial or Wonder light toast   12
2 tbsp Strawberry Preserves*   2
6 oz Sugar-Free Tang or mineral water
coffee or tea

Lunch
sliced turkey and Swiss sandwich   13
(2 oz sliced turkey, 1 oz Swiss cheese
on 2 slices Colonial or Wonder light bread
with lettuce, tomato, onion, mayo, mustard—as desired)
2 dill pickle spears
sugar-free beverage, mineral water, or tea

Snack
1 cup popcorn   5
sugar-free beverage

Supper
1 serving Cinder's Lemon Chicken*   6
1 serving Italian Zucchini Bake*   7
1 cup mixed salad greens
1 oz allowable salad dressing
sugar-free beverage, mineral water, or tea

Dessert (optional)
1 serving Elegant Kahlua Parfait*   8
Coffee

8

I've Reached My Goal, What Now?

*U*PON completion of a weight-loss regimen, any weight-loss regimen, going on a maintenance program is the dietary equivalent of the charge of the Light Brigade; it's almost doomed to failure. Of the people who reach their goal weight by dieting, almost 90 percent will regain most, if not all, of their weight within two years. Your new goal is to not contribute to this dismal statistic. If you follow the maintenance program presented in this book, you will meet your goal.

Why do people regain the weight they worked so hard to lose? Mainly because they don't understand that dieting is a lifelong undertaking. All popular fad diets and even most legitimate weight-loss programs have as their main objective the attainment of some specific goal weight. Thumb through any diet book and look at the number of pages allocated to weight loss compared to the number allocated to maintenance and you will find that most of the space is devoted to the author's particular method of losing weight. Weight loss is what sells diet books. People seem to think that there is something magical about reaching a particular weight, and that when they lose to that point, they will effortlessly remain there. Nothing is further from the truth.

I tell all of my patients on their first visit that if I could tap them on the head with a magic wand and change them instantly to their goal weight, I wouldn't be solving their problem. Thrilled though they would be to lose their excess weight instantly, they would all regain it within a year—unless they decided to alter their eating habits. If you have a weight problem, it's not going to go away just because you lose down to your goal weight—no matter how quickly you do it. It requires effort to *stay* thin. You probably know someone who is very thin yet who eats like a horse and never exercises. It's okay, I suppose, to be envious of these people, but you must realize that they are put together differently from you; they may—thanks to ancestral genes passed along—have a high rate of metabolism or some other inborn tendency that prevents them from becoming fat. You, unfortunately, don't have this ability to remain thin in the face of unlimited food consumption. Whatever genetic hookups you have that make you you are not going to change just because you're now smaller. All the biological mechanisms are still in place that caused you to be overweight in the first place, and if you return to your previous eating style, you will return to your previous weight. You must change something, and since you can't change your genetics, you must alter something over which you have some control.

What can you change? You can change the amount you exercise, the amount you eat, and you can change the types of food you eat. It seems simple enough, but as anyone who has had a weight problem knows, it is not. It's often difficult to find the time to exercise regularly, and it's extremely difficult to change eating habits over the long run. Does this mean that it is impossible to stay slim? Not really, but it does require effort. We'll devote an entire chapter later on to the exercise part of the weight maintenance equation, but now let's look at the dietary component.

Our prehistoric ancestors, who were hunters and gatherers, ate what animals they could kill as well as roots, nuts, berries, and other plant foods that were available. It required considerable expenditure of energy on their part to locate, stalk, and kill their prey, and even more to carry it back to camp. The gathering process by which they obtained their plant foods was also very energy consuming, sometimes requiring many miles of travel on foot to find, reap, and return with their forage. Most of the caloric energy they obtained from their food was probably spent in acquiring the food, so they didn't have an energy excess to be stored as fat. Today, we have just the opposite situation. We have available to us an almost infinite variety of food requiring almost no effort—other than driving to the supermarket—on our part to obtain. Our problems result from an overabundance of food rather than from a scarcity. But since good food is one of life's delights that most of us are unable or unwilling to forgo, how do we accommodate our desire for this mouthwatering fare with our desire to stay thin?

We must have a maintenance plan that will allow us to indulge our dietary vices—we're going to indulge them anyway, so why not make it part of the plan?—but still allow us to maintain our lower weight. The closer a long-term diet comes to what you want and like to eat while not dieting, the higher the probability of your sticking with it. Conversely, the further such a diet is from your pre-weight-loss eating habits, the higher the probability of failure. For example, if I could tell you that you could maintain your weight by going on a diet that would allow you to eat unlimited amounts of all the foods you love, but with the restriction that you should cut back slightly on the amount of corn you eat, you would be ecstatic because you could obviously easily stay on this hypothetical diet. Your probability of success in sticking to this diet would be high because it would require little deviation from your pre-diet eating pattern. On the other hand, if I told you that you could maintain your weight by eating nothing but two small salads, a small portion of vegetable, and 4 ounces of fish daily, you would probably not be ecstatic because you would recognize that although you would be able to maintain your weight if you stuck with this diet, your chances of sticking with it over the long haul are not good.

Let's analyze the two hypothetical diets we just discussed. The first would be a breeze to adhere to, but it would obviously not allow us to maintain our weight; while the second, although unquestionably effective, would probably be jettisoned early on because it is so restricted. We need to find a middle ground, a diet that permits us to maintain our weight, yet that requires minimal deviation from our normal diet, while providing all the necessary nutrients.

Another requirement for the ideal maintenance diet would be that it maintains or improves upon the health benefits gained from the weight-loss diet, i.e., lower blood pressure, lower serum cholesterol, stabilized blood sugar, etc.

Let's put the criteria that we have just developed for the ideal maintenance diet into tabular form so that we can refer back to it easily as we go through this chapter. The ideal maintenance diet has the following characteristics:

1. Must, if followed, maintain lower weight
2. Must be easy to stick to—realistically
3. Must provide all nutrients in required amounts
4. Must maintain or improve health

It should be obvious to you from what you have read so far that I am a champion of the low-carbohydrate/high-protein diet, and in this chapter I am going to try to convince you that it is by far the best maintenance diet. That does not mean, however, that there are no other acceptable maintenance diets. Let's use the four criteria listed above to evaluate the two most common types of maintenance diets: (1) low calorie, and (2) low carbohydrate.

Low-Calorie Diets

First, let's look at the old standby: the low-calorie diet. Low-calorie diets are typically high in complex carbohydrates and low in fat, and as we have seen, comparatively low in protein. Because many excellent sources of protein—beef, pork, and eggs, for example—are relatively high in calories, their inclusion in low-calorie diets is limited, sometimes resulting in protein deficiency. This is not to say that all low-calorie diets are protein deficient, because they are not; but often they can be, or they may require particular food combinations to provide adequate complete protein. Diets that provide most of their calories in the form of complex carbohydrates can be deficient in iron, calcium, zinc, vitamin B_{12}, and vitamin D. Fiber, which is sometimes present in large amounts in high-complex-carbohydrate diets, can interfere with the absorption of iron, calcium, zinc, and other nutrients. These deficiencies can be remedied by adding vitamin and mineral supplements to low-calorie diets to insure their nutritional adequacy.

The greatest problem I find with low-calorie diets is that they are difficult to adhere to for any length of time. There is no doubt that you can concoct a low-calorie diet that is nutritionally adequate and that will allow you to maintain your weight—if you can stick with it. Most people can't. Many dieters undergo behavior modification and other types of psychotherapeutic approaches in an effort to remain on low-calorie diets for extended periods of time. Unfortunately, most of these techniques also ultimately fail. The odds are that you have undertaken one or more low-calorie diets at some time in your past, and by virtue of the fact that you are reading this book, you have failed at successfully maintaining your weight on them. Don't feel bad, because you're not alone. Nine out of ten dieters have had your same experience and have come away from it frustrated and despairing of their lack of discipline.

Why are low-calorie diets so difficult to stick to for any length of time? Mainly because people stay hungry on them most of the time. Why do people stay hungry? Because they don't get enough to eat, and what they do eat is not very hunger satisfying. What does satisfy hunger?

Let's take a look at two ways that food satisfies hunger. First, there are nerves in the stomach that send messages to the brain when the stomach is full. If you eat a large meal that stretches your stomach, these nerves relay this information to your brain and you feel full. (The stomach-balloon procedure works in this manner. Doctors place a balloon in the patient's stomach. When this balloon is inflated, it stretches the stomach and produces a sensation of fullness.) Meals that are loaded with complex carbohydrates—the mainstay of low-calorie diets—are bulky, but they have a high water content. When they reach the stomach, they stretch the stomach wall, signaling to our brain that we are full, and we experience all the attendant feelings of fullness. But as soon as all the water in these foods is absorbed, which happens fairly quickly, we are left with a small amount of residue that is no longer bulky enough to stretch our stomachs, and we are hungry again. A good example is Oriental food, which is composed primarily of rice and other vegetables that are all high in complex carbohydrates and water; when we eat it, we experience this phenomenon of fullness followed relatively quickly by hunger. This is such a universal experience that it has given rise to many jokes on the theme of how quickly one feels hungry after eating Chinese food.

The second way in which food satisfies hunger is through hormonal feedback to the brain. In response to the consumption of fat, our intestines release hormones—cholecystokinin (CCK) and others—that act on an area of the brain that regulates our sensation of fullness or satiety. When this area of the brain—called the satiety center and located in the hypothalamus—is stimulated by CCK, we feel full irrespective of how much we've eaten. When we feel full, we stop eating. We stop eating because we are satisfied, not because we've consumed our limit of calories. Since low-calorie diets typically have a low fat content, they don't stimulate the release of much CCK and as a result, don't satisfy hunger via this hormonal feedback.

We've seen how low-calorie diets can have the potential for nutritional inadequacy, and how they fail to satisfy hunger. Let's look at another way that they can sabotage us during maintenance; they can cause adverse fluctuations in our insulin levels at critical points in our maintenance program. To better understand how these insulin-level disturbances cause problems, let's first examine the course followed by a typical dieter—see if you recognize yourself —who has lost to goal weight and is starting on a low-calorie maintenance diet.

Most dieters do fairly well in the early stages while motivation is running high, but as time goes on and motivation ebbs, they start to veer from their course. The usual train of events is for our poor dieter to struggle along on his low-calorie diet maintaining his weight until he gets into a situation such as a family reunion, surprise party, or a holiday feast in which there is a large amount of food at hand. He tries to be strong, but he finally breaks and starts shoveling food into his mouth as fast as he can. He then realizes what he has been missing, how wonderful rich food tastes, and he is off and running and usually never looks back. He starts gaining weight, and when he gains back to where he started—or more—he begins looking for the next "new" diet that will allow him to lose his weight "quickly and easily." He usually never realizes that his problem is not in losing weight, but in maintaining his lower weight. He will lose again, and again more than likely, he will try a low-calorie maintenance diet and once again, will fail.

In this dismal but all-too-common scenario, where in the train of events could our dieter have redeemed himself? He could have repented after the first debauch and started back on his maintenance diet. Had he done so, what would have happened?

Suffice it to say at this point, that when he consumed huge portions of carbohydrate-laden foods, he suffered a marked increase in blood sugar. To meet the metabolic demand of this sudden increase in blood sugar requires a high level of insulin to be released into the bloodstream, which, in turn, brings about a decrease in blood glucose levels. Sometimes, the insulin released drives the blood sugar inappropriately low. This low blood-sugar level is another one of the components of hunger. All the high-complex-carbohydrate foods available to him on his low-calorie maintenance plan have essentially this same effect: metabolizing these foods will drive his insulin level upward again, and his blood sugar down. Our errant dieter is now confronted with hunger, and he binges again.

In summary, low-calorie diets don't really fit the bill for a good maintenance diet because they fall short of fulfilling several of our standards. While low-calorie diets do allow dieters to maintain their weight if followed scrupulously, they are difficult to adhere to for any length of time because they don't sate hunger and they can make it difficult to stabilize the erratic post-overindulgence insulin levels. Also, low-calorie diets can be inadequate nutritionally, but this disadvantage can be overcome by careful preparation and food combining, or with the addition of vitamin supplements. As long as dieters get adequate nutrition and enough protein to maintain their lean-body mass, they will maintain their health with low-calorie diets, thus fulfilling the last criterion of a good maintenance diet.

Low-Carbohydrate Diets

How do low-carbohydrate diets differ from the low-calorie diets that have been shown to be so difficult to stick with? On the surface, they appear to be much the same. On one, you count calories, while on the other, you count grams of carbohydrates; one has a prescribed level of caloric intake that will allow you to maintain your weight, and the other, a level of carbohydrate intake that will allow you to maintain your weight; you can buy books to be used on one that show the number of calories in various foods, or you can buy books for the other that show the number of grams of carbohydrates in various foods. They both appear to be different versions of the same thing—diets on which you have to weigh, measure, count, and restrict your food intake. But there is one major difference—on low-calorie diets there are no free foods. All foods—and here I mean all foods that we consume for nutrition, not pure cellulose or other substances that are nonnutritive—have a certain caloric value. Granted, some foods have very few calories, but they have calories nevertheless, and these calories must be counted on low-calorie diets. Unfortunately, all these very low calorie foods have in common the property that they are not particularly filling, or they are filling only for the very short term, leaving you hungry soon after their consumption. How do low-carbohydrate diets differ?

Many foods contain *no* carbohydrates and therefore can be

eaten in virtually unlimited quantities. Remember, you're only counting carbohydrates, and foods containing no carbohydrates don't need to be counted. Beef, poultry, fish, eggs, butter, mayonnaise, any oils such as olive and canola, bouillon and broths, margarine —all contain no carbohydrates. Other foods such as cheese, heavy cream, broccoli, lettuce, mushrooms, zucchini, spinach, tofu, cucumbers, many berries, celery, cabbage, and many additional items contain few carbohydrates. These no- and low-carbohydrate foods form the backbone of our low-carbohydrate maintenance diet. How about candies, cakes, pastries, french fries, potato chips, and many other sweets and snack foods—can these be a part of a low-carbohydrate diet? No, but since they contain large numbers of calories as well as carbohydrates, neither can they be a part of a low-calorie diet. However, many items are allowed on both types of diets because they have few carbohydrates as well as few calories. Let's look at how low-carbohydrate diets fare when gauged by our rules for a good maintenance diet.

First, by following a low-carbohydrate diet, can we maintain our weight? Absolutely. It is possible to *lose* large amounts of weight on a low-carbohydrate diet, but not as quickly as with the PSMF. Remember, the PSMF is a low-carbohydrate/high-protein diet containing very few calories that allows you to lose weight rapidly, while the maintenance diet that I advocate is a low-carbohydrate/ high-protein diet containing more calories, but with a much wider range of foods. Critics of low-carbohydrate diets are always quick to point out that all the weight lost on these diets comes from fluid loss. I agree that some fluid is lost as it is on any kind of restricted diet, and probably a little more fluid is lost on low-carbohydrate diets than on others, but to say that all the weight loss comes from fluid loss is absurd. I've seen many people who have lost from 60 to 100 pounds on low-carbohydrate diets, and this weight loss could not possibly all have come from fluid loss. Anyone who has seen before and after pictures of Elizabeth Taylor can recognize that she lost much more than water, and she both lost weight and maintains her slim figure on a low-carbohydrate, high-protein diet. I can assure you that if you follow the low-carbohydrate guidelines outlined here, you will maintain your weight.

Is a low-carbohydrate diet easy to adhere to for the long run? I think that the ease with which a low-carbohydrate diet can be followed is its most important feature. It doesn't matter how good or how healthful a diet is, if you can't stick with it, it doesn't do you any good—and you can easily stick to a low-carbohydrate diet. By making small modifications in your regular pre-weight-loss diet, you can create a maintenance diet that closely approximates what you would eat if you weren't on a diet at all. And the closer a maintenance diet approximates what you ate prior to losing your weight, the higher the probability that you will stick to it. You get plenty of bulk so that your stomach wall is stretched, giving you a sensation of fullness. The fat in a low-carbohydrate diet mixes with the bulky foods and slows the passage of food from the stomach, leaving the stomach wall stretched for a longer period of time. Also, the release of CCK stimulated by this fat acts upon the brain to bring about the sensation of fullness by a different pathway. Most importantly, when you veer from your diet—as sooner or later everyone will—it is much easier to recover and get back on the maintenance regimen, which is a low-carbohydrate diet. We will devote a section of this chapter to this procedure later on, so at this time, I won't go into why this works the way it does. As you can see, the low-carbohydrate diet fulfills the requirement that a maintenance diet be easy to adhere to.

There is no doubt that you get plenty of protein on a low-carbohydrate diet, but how about other nutrients? There have been questions raised about the adequacy of calcium and some of the B vitamins on low-carbohydrate diets. If you use dairy products as part of your diet, you will get all the calcium you need. If you have a milk allergy, you can get your calcium from the vegetables used on the maintenance diet, but in some cases you may need to take calcium supplements—it depends upon your food likes and dislikes. The vegetables and fruits allowed on the maintenance diet will provide ample amounts of the B vitamins. The low-carbohydrate diet provides high amounts of iron, potassium, vitamins A, K, D, B_{12}, E, and all the trace elements and other micronutrients necessary for good health. If you eat a variety of low-carbohydrate foods, and keep your carbohydrate intake in the 60-to-90-gram-per-day range, you will easily meet or exceed all the RDAs without the need for supplements. Our third requirement for a good maintenance diet is met.

What about safety? Does a low-carbohydrate diet maintain or improve health? This is the issue that raises the hackles of many nutritionists, dieticians, and physicians. When you say the words ''low-carbohydrate diet,'' most people immediately think ''high-fat diet.'' It's a knee-jerk reaction. And since we are lambasted from all quarters with the "fact" that the high consumption of fat is bad for us, it's easy to see why these people worry. The fact is, however, *when compared to the typical Western diet, low-carbohydrate diets are also low-fat diets.* They are high-fat diets compared with typical low-calorie diets, but they are much lower in fat than the diet you ate before you lost your weight. Because unlimited portions of red meat, eggs, and other foods with a high fat content are allowed, most people jump to the conclusion that their fat intake will increase dramatically when this is simply not true. On the regular pre-weight-loss diet you were allowed unlimited quantities of these same foods—in fact, since you weren't worrying about your diet, you were allowed unlimited amounts of anything you wanted. Now, you are only permitted unlimited quantities of very few foods and must restrict or eliminate others, but in such a way that you can still have an adequate, fulfilling diet. So it stands to reason that your fat consumption would have to decrease. And if it is true that you are better off eating less fat, then you will have made an improvement by going on a low-carbohydrate diet.

When scientists tell us that the consumption of fat is bad for us, what they are saying is that the usual results of the consumption of fat are bad—total serum cholesterol and triglycerides go up, while HDL (the "good" component of cholesterol) goes down. This picture of high serum cholesterol, high triglyceride, and low HDL, to almost everyone's satisfaction, has been shown to lead to an increased incidence of heart disease. If you have been eating a diet with a low fat content and then you proceed to add a great deal of fat to this diet, in time your blood picture is probably going to change for the worse. If, however, you are already eating a diet such as the typical Western diet that is high in fat, tell me how reducing your fat intake by going on a low-carbohydrate diet is going to do anything but improve your blood picture? I have seen many studies where researchers kept subjects on an "ideal" diet with the "ideal" ratios of fat to protein to carbohydrate. After a time, the investigators obtained blood samples from these subjects and analyzed them. They then added fat to the subjects' diet, then after a time analyzed their blood again. In most, but not all, of these studies, it was apparent that the blood cholesterol levels of the subjects worsened after the addition of the fat. (Interestingly, several studies showed no significant difference.) These studies show that the *addition* of fat to the diet can be harmful, but we are not talking about an addition of fat on a low-carbohydrate diet—we are talking about a reduction of fat.

Studies that I have seen in which fat was not added to the diet but in which carbohydrates were reduced show that almost uniformly serum cholesterol decreases. In my own patients who have lowered their cholesterol on the PSMF, I have found a maintenance of this lower cholesterol on the low-carbohydrate maintenance diet to be the rule.

There are other reasons besides the fact that they are lower in fat that low-carbohydrate diets decrease serum cholesterol—for one, they decrease the synthesis of cholesterol. We will discuss these reasons in greater detail in a later chapter. But for now, I want to make sure that you understand that low-carbohydrate diets are *not* high-fat diets, and that not only are they not a hazard to your health, they are very beneficial.

Low-carbohydrate diets allow you to maintain your weight, are easily adhered to, provide all the nutrients in adequate amounts, and improve your health. They are the ideal maintenance diet, fulfilling all our requirements. Before we go over the low-carbohydrate maintenance regimen, let's look at a new way of counting carbohydrates that gives us an even wider range of foods to choose from.

Counting Carbohydrates: A Better Method

In previous books or articles you may have read giving instructions on carbohydrate counting, you were told to get a book listing the carbohydrate content of various foods, and then to select for your diet those foods—low in carbohydrates—the carbohydrate values of which, when totaled, equaled your day's allotment. If you kept your intake of carbohydrates below some specified maximum, you would either lose or maintain your weight depending upon your goal and the number of carbohydrates permitted—usually few if you were trying to lose, more if you were just trying to maintain. If you followed a low-carbohydrate diet, you noticed that many things you loved to eat were crawling with carbohydrates and were therefore not permitted—or were permitted only in small amounts. But you can now expand your carbohydrate horizons in varying amounts and allow yourself to eat many more foods than before because of the new way in which dietary fiber is measured.

The total carbohydrate content of foods as listed on the label is a combination of sugars, starches, and fiber. Only the sugars and starches actually count as carbohydrates, because we cannot digest the fiber. Only the nonfiber portion of the carbohydrate need be counted. Previously, the only fiber that could be detected in foods was the so-called crude fiber, which was measured by very "crude" methods indeed. The amount of "crude fiber" found in most foods was so insignificant that it was not even worth listing. Now, food chemists measure fiber using different methods that give results that closely approximate the actual fiber content of the food in question. The fiber content of foods as determined by these newer methods is listed as "dietary fiber," and in many cases it is substantial.

When you start to count carbohydrates, subtract the amount of fiber from the total carbohydrate content of the food, and you will be left with the amount of carbohydrate that actually figures into your diet. Let's refer to this carbohydrate—the sugar and starch portion only—that your body can actually digest as the "effective carbohydrate content" (ECC) of the food you are measuring. Since your body doesn't treat fiber as it does carbohydrate, there is no reason to measure it. How does this business of the ECC actually work in practice? Let's look at an example.

Two cups of fresh, steamed broccoli—a substantial serving— contain 15.9 grams of total carbohydrate and would take a pretty good bite out of a day's 60-gram quota, but only 4.2 grams of this carbohydrate are digestible and must be counted—the other 11.7 grams are fiber. By this reckoning, you will have 55.8 grams of carbohydrate remaining that you can eat instead of the 44.1 grams you would have had, had you counted total carbohydrate—a significant difference. How about cauliflower? Two cups of cauliflower contain 10.7 grams of carbohydrate of which 4.2 grams are fiber, leaving 6.5 grams of ECC—not quite as good a carbohydrate bargain as broccoli, but almost. By following this method, you will be able to add many vegetables and a fair number of fruits to your diet without going over your carbohydrate limit. At the same time, you will be selecting items high in fiber that will improve your health in many ways, as we will discuss in Chapter 10.

A problem inherent in following this method arises from the fact that few books list the "dietary fiber" content of foods—most, if they list it at all, list "crude fiber," which is a falsely low figure. For example, broccoli has a "crude fiber" content of only 3.7 grams per two cups rather than the 11.7 mentioned above. By using this "crude fiber" figure, you would err on the side of limiting your carbohydrate intake rather than in overindulging, and you would continue to maintain your weight. But why be limited if it is not necessary? I have included a list of the ECC of several fruits and vegetables along with their total carbohydrate and fiber content in Appendix C. I hope that someone will publish a more extensive list of foods and their dietary fiber content in the near future.

You will be surprised to see that some foods that you may have thought to be high in fiber are actually not. Popcorn, for instance. Almost everyone seems to think that popcorn is loaded with fiber —probably because it feels "fibery" or crunchy in the mouth. I've seen popcorn referred to as "nature's broom," meaning of course that its high fiber content helps to "sweep" the colon clean. Three cups of popcorn—a typical serving—contain 14.4 grams of carbohydrate, but only 1.2 grams of fiber, resulting in an ECC of 13.2 grams. You would have to eat almost 30 cups of popcorn to get the same amount of fiber as you would get from 2 cups of steamed broccoli. Lettuce is another food that almost everyone thinks of as fiber rich. I don't know how many times I've heard the statement "I get plenty of fiber; I eat a large salad every day." Let's assume that a large salad is three cups of lettuce. How much fiber is really there? Three cups of lettuce provide approximately 3.5 grams of total carbohydrate and only 1.8 grams of fiber—not plenty, that's for sure, when you consider that most sources recommend at least 25 grams per day. Again, there is as much fiber in 2 cups of broccoli as in almost 20 cups of lettuce. The lesson to be learned from these examples is to not assume to know the fiber or carbohydrate content of foods—look them up either in Appendix C or one of the many books available that lists the carbohydrate content of foods. But be careful, because most of these books don't provide values for fiber. Sometimes, when they do provide values for fiber, these figures will be given for crude fiber, a value that is way too low for our ECC calculation purposes. If a particular book does not state that its fiber values are calculated as *dietary* fiber, compare the figures in that reference book for a particular fruit or vegetable to those you find listed in my own Appendix C. If the values are similar, the reference book is using dietary fiber, and the figures may be used in ECC calculations. On the other hand, if the fiber values in the reference book are considerably lower than those in Appendix C, the reference book is using crude fiber calculations, which are far too low for accurate ECC calculations.

As you proceed with the maintenance diet, if you will use this method of carbohydrate counting, you will be able to enjoy a wide variety of foods in quantities unimagined by previous carbohydrate counters. By selecting foods with a low ECC, you will tend toward those foods that are high in fiber and will thus negate another criticism of low-carbohydrate diets—that they are fiber deficient.

Maintenance Diet Protocols

At this point, as discussed at the end of Chapter 7, you should have established the carbohydrate intake that will start you on your maintenance path. It will be about 60 grams per day—or higher if you are still in ketosis on 60 grams per day. Whichever it is, that is your "rough" maintenance carbohydrate intake level, and your starting point. While remaining at this level, you may continue to lose weight slowly, or you may instead gain slowly, but probably you will maintain your weight. If you maintain your weight, this becomes your long-term maintenance level of carbohydrate intake, but if you continue to either gain or lose weight, you must fine-tune your diet. You do this by either adding or subtracting carbohydrate from your diet until your weight stabilizes: adding if you are losing weight, subtracting if you are gaining. You should add to or decrease your carbohydrate intake in 10-gram increments. If, for example, you start at 60 grams per day and continue to lose, you would increase your intake of carbohydrates to 70 grams per day and remain at that level for a week and watch what happens. If your weight stabilizes, remain there; if you continue to lose, go up to 80 grams per day. Continue to manipulate your carbohydrate intake in this manner, remaining for a week at each 10-gram incremental level, until your weight stabilizes. You will then have determined the amount of carbohydrate that you can consume daily and still maintain your weight.

In the several thousand patients that I have put through this regimen, I have found the outside limits of carbohydrate intake to be from 40 grams per day to 130 grams per day. The vast majority of my patients, however, have fallen in the range of from 50 to 70 grams per day. Once you have determined your maintenance carbohydrate intake level (MCL), you limit your carbohydrate intake to that amount daily, while eating virtually unlimited amounts of non-carbohydrate-containing foods. And remember, when you're counting carbohydrates, count ECCs and not total carbohydrates.

As long as your weight remains where you want it, you can remain at this MCL. If your weight starts to shift in either direction—and you have been adhering to your maintenance diet—then you should again adjust your MCL as described above, but this should not happen often, if at all.

Now that you have identified your MCL, which let's say for example is 60 grams per day, you can launch into the heart of your maintenance diet—your lifelong eating plan. You can prepare many low-carbohydrate meals from the recipes in Chapter 9, and you can prepare many more by using the low-ECC foods listed in Appendix C. You will find that with a little inventiveness you will be able to modify many of your favorite recipes to make them fit into your maintenance guidelines. The beauty of this maintenance diet is in its simplicity. It allows you a wide range of foods—foods that you can select based on your taste preferences—from which to choose, with the only restriction being that you keep your carbohydrate intake at or below your MCL. That's it—no other rules. What about fat, can you have all the fat you want? Theoretically, yes, but in actuality you will eat much less fat than before. Let me explain.

Many foods that are loaded with carbohydrates are also loaded with fat. Doughnuts, pastries of all kinds, french fries, ice cream, milkshakes, many breads, pancakes, waffles, potato salad, candies —all, and others too numerous to mention, are high in fat as well as high in carbohydrate content. When you eliminate these from your diet in order to keep your carbohydrate intake within bounds, you will automatically eliminate a large amount of fat as well. If you add some butter or cheese to your vegetables because it makes them taste better, or if you eat red meat or eggs, it doesn't really matter because you will have already eliminated so much fat from your diet by staying within your carbohydrate limit. Other than the obvious things that you would probably do anyway, such as trimming excess fat from your steaks before grilling and not floating everything you cook on lard, you don't have to pay much attention to the fat that you eat because it is reduced simultaneously as you reduce carbohydrates. Compared to the average American diet, *low-carbohydrate diets are low-fat diets*. If you take care of your carbohydrate intake, your fat intake will take care of itself.

Is that all there is to maintenance? If I just keep my carbohydrate intake at or below my MCL, will I always maintain my weight? It sounds too simple. It is simple, and it is easy—especially if you don't like doughnuts, pastries, candies, Mom's apple pie, and a host of other carbohydrate-laden delicacies. But what if you do? It's a "piece of cake" to stay on a low-carbohydrate diet if you don't crave carbohydrates. But what if you do crave them? Then, it's not quite so simple. If you plan on maintaining your lower weight, you must work at it. It requires of you some effort and restraint. Chapter 14, on discipline, will help you deal with your situation by instructing you in how to take control, but there is a dietary modification that will also help. I'm referring to the dietary "vacations" and subsequent recovery periods we discussed earlier. Let's look at how this works.

First, let me state that you will probably be healthier if you stick to your low-carbohydrate diet without indiscretion for the rest of your life. (Not only would you be healthier, you would probably be a candidate for sainthood.) Questions of good health notwithstanding, my best efforts (or anyone's best efforts, for that matter) are not going to keep you from eating foods high in carbohydrates for the rest of your life. These foods taste too good and are too easily available. (Our early ancestors, if they wanted to partake of the only refined sweet available to them, had to knock a beehive out of a tree and brave a swarm of irate bees—a far cry from driving down to the local ice cream parlor for a banana split.) So, let's be realistic; you're going to eat sweets and starches from time to time irrespective of your best intentions. If you're going to do this—and you will—how can we work it into your maintenance diet? What will it do to your health?

You can deal with this lust for carbohydrates that we all seem to be afflicted with by taking breaks from your regular maintenance diet: breaks in which you indulge in all the carbohydrates you want. These breaks should be planned for and spaced *at least* three weeks apart. I encourage my patients to take them over long weekends, on their vacations from work, on Super Bowl weekend, during family get-togethers, and any times that they would normally be tempted to veer from their diet. During these breaks, you should eat anything and everything you want. Eat all the things you've been craving. You'll feel lousy after you've done this, and if you had symptoms of gastric reflux, heartburn, or feelings of bloating before you started your low-carbohydrate regimen, they will probably return—but only temporarily. (If nothing else, this will convince you of the merits of a low-carbohydrate diet.) After one of these debauches, you will be ready to go back on your maintenance diet. You will do so swearing never to repeat the experience again —but don't worry, that feeling will pass, and before you know it, you'll again be craving a cheese Danish. After you complete one of these little dietary vacations you must recover from it.

You may need to recover from a faint as well when you step on the scales after an overindulgence of carbohydrates. You will gain from 4 to 8 pounds very quickly. Unbelievably quickly. But it will all be from fluid retention. While you are on the maintenance diet, your blood insulin levels will be low. As well as regulating the levels of glucose in your blood, insulin has the property of causing the kidneys to retain sodium and water. If your insulin levels fall —as they do on low-carbohydrate diets—your kidneys release the sodium and water, causing you to urinate more frequently. This increased water release or diuresis is what causes so much weight to be lost so early on low-carbohydrate diets. It is also what reduces high blood pressure. The reverse takes place when one who has been on a low-carbohydrate diet binges on carbohydrates. First, blood-sugar levels go up, followed by a rise in the level of insulin, and then the kidneys start to retain fluid. As you retain fluid, you gain weight. To reverse this weight gain, all you must do is to go on a diet very restricted in carbohydrates for two or three days— just long enough to lose the excess fluid you put on.

This "recovery" diet is the same one you used when you started eating again after the PSMF. It is described on page 119. It provides only 20 grams of carbohydrate daily and will rapidly lower your insulin levels, which will allow your kidneys to jettison the excess fluid you have retained. After you have lost back to your ideal weight, go back to your maintenance level of carbohydrate intake and continue from there.

Your maintenance regimen from this point on should be stretches of time during which you carefully adhere to your MCL punctuated with occasional dietary vacations and recoveries. If you follow this plan, you will maintain your weight while at the same time allowing yourself to indulge *occasionally* in anything you want. It is a reasonable, realistic approach to weight maintenance. We asked earlier if this is a healthy way to maintain. As I said, it's probably not as healthful as rigidly adhering to the diet, but what about the alternative? If you don't adhere to the diet, and don't have a plan for that contingency, what happens? You start eating nonstop and regain your weight. I think that it is infinitely more healthful to maintain your lower weight while occasionally debauching than it is to regain your weight while trying to diet. I am a firm believer in the fact that you will be more inclined to deny yourself rich, sweet foods today if you know that you can have all of them you want next weekend. If you think that you can never have a doughnut again, you will be much more likely to reach for one now. With the knowledge that you can indulge in your favorite foods, and with a plan for doing so without fear of gaining weight, you can look forward to a lifetime of being slim without a lifetime of sacrifice and denial.

9

Living High the Low-Carbohydrate Way

*I*F you are now near your goal weight and beginning the transition process from the PSMF to a full-food diet, you are ready to begin a lifetime of low-carbohydrate cooking and eating. While in the weight-loss phase, you may already have begun thinking of food in terms of carbohydrate content, and if so, then you are that much ahead. I cannot stress strongly enough at this point that if you have *not* begun to think carbohydrate content, you must now reorient your thinking, because in your smooth transition to maintenance, the carbohydrate content of foods assumes a new importance—you must think carbohydrates, not merely calories.

As we discussed in Chapter 8, the beauty of a controlled-carbohydrate lifestyle is its richness. So many foods that are sinfully rich, deliciously satisfying, and even high in calories have zero or very few carbohydrates. But learning to control daily carbohydrate intake—to maintain your hard-won goal—will be a lifelong process. And unfortunately for most of us, adhering to any maintenance plan will not be an easy proposition.

There are two reasons that make it difficult for Americans to stay on any kind of long-term diet, be it this or any other maintenance regimen: (1) we are a society of nibblers, and (2) we are a society that eats on the run. Both of these problems mean that we eat a lot of junk food and/or fast food. If we can overcome these obstacles, we are well on our way to successful weight control. The obvious way to overcome them is to forsake them—but that method is not in keeping with our policy of being realistic. How can we deal with this situation successfully on a low-carbohydrate maintenance diet? Let's look first at the problem of nibbling.

What do we nibble and snack on while we watch television or read? What do we serve when we entertain casually? What do we eat at cocktail parties? What do we eat at restaurants before the food is served? Hors d'oeuvres. All kinds of chips—potato chips, corn chips, taco chips, etc. Crackers of many different varieties. And of course, what would the chips and crackers be without dips? There are bean dips, sour-cream-based dips, guacamole dips, cheese dips, mayonnaise-based dips, yogurt-based dips, tomato-based dips such as salsa, and many others. Along with the chips and crackers, we use carrots, broccoli, celery, and other crudités to scoop our dip. We love cupcakes, brownies, cookies, doughnuts, and pastries—all kinds of bakery goods. And let's not forget candy—candy bars, fudge, mints, hard candy, suckers, candy corn, expensive gift chocolates, the list is endless. There are even those little, nasty, almost tasteless, stick-to-your-teeth, rubbery, shaped-in-the-image-of-animals candies, the kind my children eat in unbelievable quantities whenever parental surveillance is lax. The list lengthens and we haven't even mentioned ice cream bars, Popsicles, Fudgesicles, and a host of others. The point of all this is to make you aware that these are *not* food—these are snacks. We eat these in addition to the "three squares" that we get every day—we don't need any of these things to be adequately nourished.

But need them or not, as a rule, we seem to be driven to snack. Why? Is the basis for our obsession with snacks and sweets that we are afflicted with a National Sweet Tooth? One could certainly make that case.

How many times have you heard someone say, "I'm a sweet-aholic?" Or, "I crave sweets." You may even consider yourself a "sweetaholic" in that you love to eat sweet, sugary foods—but is it really the sweet that you crave? Do you often eat sugar by the spoonful? I doubt that you do. What you actually crave is the combination of sugar *and* fat. And almost all the foods we consider to be "sweets"—candy, pastries, fudge, cake, malts, ice cream, and many, many others—are, in fact, this fat-sugar combination. Even items not generally thought of as being sweet are also combinations of fat and carbohydrate. Potato chips, corn chips, and french fries are three that quickly come to mind. We even make our own combinations of fat and carbohydrate. I've never known anyone who eats butter by itself, but many people combine it with bread, potatoes, corn, popcorn, and many other starchy, carbohydrate-laden foods. By way of example, let's look at the potato a little more closely. A baked potato is a starchy vegetable that contains a large amount of carbohydrate but no fat. But how do most people eat baked potatoes? They fill them with butter or sour cream or cheese sauce or even a combination of these. It's the combination that's tasty. Of the two items in the fat-sugar equation, I don't know why sugar got the bum rap—why isn't anyone ever a "fataholic"?

In the previous chapter we discussed the fact that a low-carbohydrate diet is much lower in fat than most people suppose. The major reason for that is this fat-sugar combination we love so much. When we decrease our intake of carbohydrates, we invariably decrease our intake of the fat that so often accompanies it. About the only instances in which we take in large amounts of sugar without the fat are when we drink soft drinks or other sweetened beverages. We sometimes use sugar in coffee and tea, but again many people add fat in the form of cream. In terms of a low-carbohydrate diet, the use of sugar as a sweetener in beverages has pretty much been replaced by various noncarbohydrate sweeteners, but we still don't have available an artificial fat. (Let me digress just a moment on the subject of artificial sweeteners; I feel that Equal or Nutrasweet—the generic name is aspartame—is a very safe substance. It has undergone more rigid analysis by a multitude of agencies than any substance in recent times and has been found to cause very few problems. I would think that it probably causes fewer problems than the sugar it replaces.)

As far as nibbling and snacking go, what *can* we eat on a low-carbohydrate maintenance program? Some snack foods are fine on the maintenance diet, and if we stick to the right ones, we need not feel deprived. Granted, it takes some restraint to limit ourselves to the allowable snacks, but the payoff—remaining slim—more than compensates.

What are the allowable snacks? Those that contain little or no carbohydrate. This chapter, in the recipe section, describes several candies that are low in carbohydrate and are acceptable—but remember, even though low relative to regular candies, these snacks do contain some carbohydrate that you must count. Most dips—cheese, sour cream, and others—are acceptable. The problem with dips, however, lies with the dipping instrument. Virtually all crackers and chips contain carbohydrates, and even though they don't contain much per chip or cracker, when eaten by the handful, the carbohydrates add up. You may use raw vegetable crudités, which have few carbohydrates and significantly more fiber, or pork rinds, which have none. Pork rinds are light, expanded, air-filled pieces of pork skin that are crunchy, chiplike, and have their own unique taste. They can be used instead of chips and crackers to scoop the various dips, and most people find them quite tasty. They contain no carbohydrates. Even though pork rinds are 100 percent fat, I doubt that they contain much more fat than an equivalent weight of potato or corn chips, but unlike potato or corn chips, they have no carbohydrates, which is to our advantage. So, you can use pork rinds or fresh vegetable crudités and various dips for snacks. Don't forget, however, to count the carbohydrates in the dip—sour-cream dips, for instance, contain about eight grams per cup.

You can snack on all kinds of hors d'oeuvres made primarily of meat such as chicken wings, meatballs, boiled shrimp, and many others (see recipe section). Cheeses of all kinds—except the sweetened ones, of course—are acceptable to snack on. Most cheeses contain only one gram of carbohydrate per ounce. I have included several recipes in this chapter for foods that can be nibbled and snacked on, but they do require some preparation. You can't just open a bag or tear off a wrapper and start stuffing your mouth.

This leads me to the second problem we all have, namely, that we often eat on the run or don't want to wait to have food prepared that is more healthful. In fact, we often don't even want to wait to have food that is more tasty. Think of the small "mom-and-pop" hamburger stands that you used to see everywhere. You would go up to the window and have your order taken and usually be given a number and told that you would be called when your burger was ready. The food was uniformly good, the burgers were thick and juicy, but it took a few minutes to prepare them. Now, all these places, except in the smallest towns, are being replaced by the franchise-chain fast-food outlets. The requirement for survival is no longer how good the food is, but how quickly it can be served. Almost everyone, as they're chewing on a tasteless offering from the local chain fast-food place, laments the passing of the old home-cooked-hamburger places and reminisces about the superior flavor and quality they provided. I'm not trying to point a finger at anyone for this, I've done it myself many times. I've sacrificed quality for quickness. And I see the trend developing in which people spend less and less effort on obtaining their food—whatever is the easiest is best.

Look at the increasing prevalence of drive-through windows. The first time I saw one of these was in California twenty years ago, and you had to suffer the indignity of giving your order to a jack-in-the-box. Now, practically every fast-food place has a drive-through window. The thing that never ceases to amaze me about these drive-through windows is how long people are willing to wait to avoid having to make the effort to get out of their cars and walk in. Often I have seen a whole string of cars in the drive-through line and not a person inside at the counter. You could park your car, walk in, order, get your order, walk back out, get in your car and drive away, and still be way ahead of the people in the drive-through line. Home delivery of food is on the rise. Five years ago in Little Rock, you had to go out for pizza; now every pizza place, almost without exception, delivers. As a part of their advertising, they stress how quickly they can have the hot pizza in your hands—they even offer rebates if they aren't speedy enough. What does all this have to do with the maintenance plan? Nothing other than to once again point out the two greatest obstacles facing anyone about to embark upon a lifetime program of weight maintenance: snacking and sacrificing quality for speed in the preparation of food.

I can practically guarantee you that the faster the food, the more fat and carbohydrates it contains. If you want to do well and be successful on your maintenance diet, you are going to have to be willing to spend some time on food preparation. Many of the recipes described in this chapter can be prepared in an amount of time equal to or smaller than that needed to get in your car and drive to the local fast-food outlet, pick up your order at the drive-through window, drive home, take it out of the bag, and serve it. And amazingly, many of these same recipes can be prepared at much less expense than an equivalent amount of fast food. Which do you suppose would taste better?

It would be unrealistic to expect to prepare every meal at home, to never dine out at a restaurant or eat fast food again. It's just too much a part of our culture, and often we find ourselves in situations where eating a fast-food hamburger, chicken breast, or pizza is practically unavoidable. What do we do then?

Maintenance on the Run

As we discussed in Chapter 6, dining away from home does not have to be a dietary disaster during the PSMF, nor does it on maintenance. In fast-food establishments, you must learn to be selective. Choose such menu items as a double-patty burger and remove the bun, or have a salad from the salad bar, or a bowl of chili (the beans run the carbohydrate content of these chilis up quite a bit, so be careful). Even fried chicken or a chicken breast sandwich (if you remove the bun) has relatively few carbohydrates. Fried items do have a much higher fat content, however, and you must bear that in mind. Steer clear of the baked potatoes, french fries, fried pies, sundaes and shakes, and all nondiet beverages. As far as condiments go, mustard and mayonnaise have no carbohydrates, but be careful with catsup—it has 4 grams per tablespoon. Most restaurants will offer selections that with minor modifications on your part will allow you to stay well within your daily carbohydrate allotment.

Let's look at a specific example of how this works. At a popular fast-food chain restaurant, if you have a typical meal consisting of a bacon cheeseburger, french fries, and soft drink, you will be consuming about 96 grams of carbohydrate and 42 grams of fat. By removing the bun and eating your bacon cheeseburger with a fork, forgoing the french fries, and having a diet soft drink, you can eliminate about 94 grams of carbohydrate and almost 20 grams of fat. (The 20 grams of fat eliminated comes from that in the bun and the french fries, and it doesn't include the 5–10 grams absorbed from the meat patty by the bun. The first time you do this bun-jettisoning maneuver, notice how soaked with fat the bun on the bottom of the burger is.) I'm not trying to encourage you to eat like this all the time, I'm just pointing out that, with a little modification, meals at fast-food chains can be worked into your maintenance program.

If your dining excursion takes you to a somewhat nicer spot, have no fear. When the menu arrives, search for meat, chicken, fish, or seafood entrées that are broiled, baked, grilled, or even very lightly breaded and sautéed. Even items such as veal medallions in a cream sauce will be low enough in carbohydrate content to be acceptable on maintenance. Remember, we are counting carbohydrates, not calories. Often, the entrée will be accompanied by a sauté of carrots, zucchini, broccoli, or green beans. Perfect! If, however, the vegetable selection is potatoes in any form or pasta, you must take great care to use restraint. A single side-dish serving of, for example, fettucini carries a 17-to-20-gram-carbohydrate price tag, and a baked potato as many as 50 grams. For many people, 50 grams may wipe out nearly the whole day's maintenance allotment. Here is where your restraint must win out. If you want the potato, have it, but account for it by "recovering" for a day or two. Better yet, cut the potato in half and reduce your carbohydrate load to only 25. I urge you to place yourself beyond temptation if you feel your resolve weakening. Remove the rest from your sight; wrap it in a napkin; ask the waiter for a doggie bag. The same premise holds true for breads. If the waiter brings a delicious hard roll and butter, have one; the cost in carbohydrates will be about 18 to 20 grams, and that's fine as long as you account for it in your daily allotment. When the dessert menu arrives, look for good carbohydrate values: items such as strawberries Romanoff, fresh berries and cream, melon, custards, or specialty coffees, for example. Keeping track of your daily carbohydrate load will take a little extra effort at first, but with time, the counting becomes second nature.

Cooking and Dining at Home

My patients, my staff, and I have searched out the recipes contained in this chapter and have modified them in such a way that from soup to nuts, they are low in carbohydrates. I have calculated and listed the carbohydrate, protein, fat, fiber, and calorie content for each of them at the end of the recipe. I have selected recipes that I feel will be certain to please all palates and will provide you with a wide dietary variety—I promised you earlier that this diet would not be boring.

One of the mainstays of a low-carbohydrate diet is meat of many varieties. Aside from the various recipes presented in this chapter, meats of all kinds may simply be grilled over charcoal. In response to consumer demand for red meats with a reduced fat content, the USDA has come up with a new category for the grading of meat—Select. Previously, the higher the USDA grading, the higher the fat content, with Prime being the highest in fat of all. Now, when you choose Select beef, you get a cut that contains about 25 percent less fat. But if you choose a different cut of beef than Select, you should remove all the visible fat before grilling. Whether it is a Select grade or another trimmed of fat before cooking, as far as I'm concerned, nothing beats a grilled steak, large salad with an olive oil dressing, and a cooked green vegetable for a low-carbohydrate feast.

Despite being able to eat steaks and other rich foods that are low in carbohydrate, most people miss breads and other foods containing large amounts of flour. Since refined wheat flour has a high carbohydrate content—from 80 to 110 grams per cup—products containing it cannot be eaten in much quantity on the maintenance diet. Fortunately, due to the development of a new product, this is starting to change for the better.

Flour of the Future

Because of its unique properties, flour has been used for centuries in the baking of bread, as a thickening agent in gravies and sauces, and for a multitude of purposes in many other foods. And consequently, any foods containing large amounts of flour also contain a corresponding amount of carbohydrate. Recently a product —microcrystalline cellulose—has been developed to the point that it can be produced in large quantities. This cellulose product—its trade name is Solka Floc—is made from wood. As we discussed in Chapter 3, cellulose is fiber in its most basic form, and whether it comes from wood or from green beans, our bodies respond to it in the same way—they pass it through undigested. Solka Floc is a white powder that looks like flour and is odorless and tasteless. It can be used in many recipes calling for flour in place of a portion of the flour—sometimes up to one-third. It can be used as a thickening agent in sauces and has many other uses as well. And since it isn't digestible, it doesn't have to be counted in carbohydrate-counting plans. Of the many "light" breads available, all use Solka Floc or similar products to replace a portion of the flour. Currently, Colonial Light Bread is the brand that contains the least actual digestible carbohydrate. The label states that this bread contains 9 grams of carbohydrate per slice, but of these 9 grams, 3 are Solka Floc, leaving an Effective Carbohydrate Content of 6 grams per slice. Some other brands of "light" bread have an ECC of 7. More and more food manufacturers are starting to use Solka Floc in their products in place of some of the flour and cornstarch, but at this point it is available commercially in large amounts and only by mail order in small amounts.

Aside from not being readily available, Solka Floc is a little bit tricky to cook with. You can't just substitute it for flour in a particular proportion and cook away—you have to approach it a little differently. William Parker of Memphis, who is a retired restaurateur, a recipe developer, and a long-time low-carbohydrate dieter, became enamored of the properties of Solka Floc and its application to low-carbohydrate dieting. In his test kitchen, he has developed many delicious recipes using Solka Floc in many different ways in low-carbohydrate cooking. He has privately published a cookbook that describes in detail the exact way to use this product to produce great results. His book also contains many wonderful low-carbohydrate recipes—some of which he has permitted me to use in the recipe section in this book—that don't require the use of Solka Floc. I highly recommend his cookbook, and you can get it by sending $4.95 plus $1.50 for postage and handling to:

> William Mark Parker
> Delicious Low-Carbohydrate Recipes
> 6055 Primacy Parkway, Suite 401
> Memphis, TN 38119

Mr. Parker has also started packaging Solka Floc in noncommercial amounts and will send you information on the mail-order purchase of this product along with the cookbook.

With the recipes in this book, in other low-carbohydrate cookbooks such as Mr. Parker's, and of your own development, you will become expert at controlled-carbohydrate cooking and eating. When you hear "Duncan Hines chocolate chip cookie," you will think "Seven grams of carbohydrate each (not to mention almost 3 grams of fat)." Quickly, you will learn which foods have few carbohydrates and which are dietary thieves: foods that steal your entire day's allotment in one fell swoop. You will find yourself doing mental arithmetic automatically as you keep a running total of your carbohydrate gram intake through the day. You will soon be creating your own recipes as cooking with carbohydrate content in mind becomes second nature to you.

Keeping control of your daily carbohydrate intake will be a simple undertaking as long as you follow the guidelines of the maintenance chapter and utilize the foods and recipes provided. Until keeping a mental tab of your daily intake of carbohydrate grams *does* become second nature, you may want to keep track in a diary or table.

With these guidelines and the recipes that follow, you should be able to dine out or at home without piling on excess carbohydrates and pounds. Just remember, limit your snacking to low-carbohydrate items, and try to take the time to prepare your foods, and you will be way, way ahead of the weight-maintenance game. *Bon appétit!*

The Recipes

Egg Dishes

Kaye's Quiche

. . . . Kaye, one of our nurses and a veteran low-carbohydrate dieter, brought this delicious crustless quiche to work as a leftover for lunch. The taste is superb, the first day or the next.

Ahead of time, THAW
10 oz. pkg frozen chopped spinach.
PRESS all excess water from spinach.

In a skillet:
MELT   *1 tbsp butter*
SAUTÉ   *3 tbsp minced raw onion until clear*
Set aside.
COOK and CRUMBLE   *4 slices bacon, crisp*
In a mixing bowl:
BEAT   *5 eggs*
ADD   *spinach, bacon, and onion*
POUR mixture into quiche pan sprayed with no-stick cooking
    spray.
BAKE at 350° for 30 to 35 minutes.

Serves 6.

Nutritional Values per Serving

Carbohydrate	3.1 gms
Protein	14.6 gms
Calories	226
Fat	17.4 gms
Fiber	1.0 gms

Delightfully Devilish Eggs

. . . . when all the kids are home, we have to double the recipe because they can eat these eggs faster than we can make them.

HARD-BOIL   *6 large eggs*
PEEL and SLICE in halves.
REMOVE yolks to a bowl, SET whites aside.
MASH the yolks with a fork.
To the mashed yolks:
ADD   *¼ cup salmon, drained and boned*
                  ¼ cup softened cream cheese
                  ¼ tsp garlic powder
                  Salt and pepper to taste
BEAT mixture until smooth.
STUFF egg-white halves with mixture.
GARNISH with   *a sprinkle of caviar or*
                    a few capers or
                    a slice of black olive if desired

Serves 6.

Nutritional Values per Serving

Carbohydrate	0.5 gms
Protein	4.4 gms
Calories	63
Fat	4.8 gms
Fiber	0.0 gms

Breakfast Extravaganza

. . . . my own creation, devised long before the advent of my diet program, is tailor-made for the program. The eggplant adds a new dimension to scrambled eggs.

In a large skillet:

MELT	*2 tbsp butter*
SAUTÉ	*½ white onion, chopped*
	1 tsp minced garlic until transparent
ADD to skillet	*½ eggplant, peeled and diced*
	¼ cup chopped fresh bell pepper
	¼ cup chopped fresh mushrooms

SAUTÉ all until just done.

In a mixing bowl:

BEAT	*8 eggs until frothy*
BEAT IN	*1 tsp black pepper*
	1 tsp Original Herb Seasoning
	1 tsp salt

POUR egg mixture into skillet with sautéed vegetables.
GENTLY lift mixture with large spoon to mix and cook.

Serves 4.

Nutritional Values per Serving

Carbohydrate	5.2 gms
Protein	12.9 gms
Calories	230
Fat	17.4 gms
Fiber	1.3 gms

Casserole Egg-Stravaganza

. . . . Sunday brunch at the Eades' household is a tradition. This egg casserole has been served at the brunch to our family and friends for years, and always to rave reviews.

SPRAY a 2-qt casserole dish with no-stick cooking spray.
DICE   *6 pieces raw bacon into casserole dish*
MICROWAVE on high 2–3 minutes (until just done).
In a mixing bowl:
BEAT   *12 eggs*
GRATE   *4 oz hot Monterey Jack cheese into eggs*
ADD   *Salt, pepper, and Original Herb Seasoning to taste*
POUR egg mixture into casserole with bacon.
MICROWAVE covered on high 3 minutes, STIR, continue
        microwaving another 2 minutes on high. STIR again and
        check for doneness. Continue microwaving on high for 30
        seconds at a time, stirring between, until done to your taste.

Serves 6.

Nutritional Values per Serving

Carbohydrate	1.6 gms
Protein	18.7 gms
Calories	265
Fat	19.9 gms
Fiber	0.1 gms

Swiss Egg Casserole

. . . . *elegant and rich for romantic midnight buffet breakfasts or prepared in multiples, for your own version of the Sunday brunch.*

PREHEAT oven to 400°.
SPRAY a baking dish with no-stick cooking spray.
LINE the bottom with *2 oz Swiss cheese slices.*
In a separate bowl:
BEAT   *4 eggs*
ADD   *⅛ tsp nutmeg*
                  ⅛ tsp caraway seeds
                  ½ tsp Krazy Mixed-up Salt
POUR into baking dish.
TOP with   *2 more oz Swiss cheese slices*
DOT with   *2 tbsp butter*
POUR on   *¼ cup heavy cream*
SPRINKLE on   *dash pepper*
BAKE at 400° for 15 minutes.

Serves 2.

Nutritional Values per Serving

Carbohydrate	4.5 gms
Protein	29.1 gms
Calories	545
Fat	45.0 gms
Fiber	0.1 gms.

Egg Salad

. . . . makes delicious sandwiches on Colonial light toast or bread, and prepared in quantity, makes an elegant hors d'oeuvre on crackers, toasted bread rounds, or with pork rinds at cocktail buffets.

HARDBOIL   *8 eggs*

COOL quickly under running water, refrigerate.

PEEL and CHOP   *the eggs*

ADD   *2 tbsp chopped black olives*
                     1 tsp minced onion
                     ½ tsp garlic powder
                     1 tbsp chopped dill pickle
                     2 tbsp real mayonnaise
                     1 tbsp Dijon-style mustard

MIX well.

Serves 4 as sandwiches.

Nutritional Values per Serving

Carbohydrate	1.9 gms
Protein	12.4 gms
Calories	215
Fat	17.1 gms
Fiber	0.1 gms

Meat, Fish, and Fowl

Rosemary Chicken

. . . . a graduate-school friend once prepared this dish for me. Over the years, it has become a staple around our supper table.

WASH and SEASON
4 medium-sized chicken breast halves (about 2 lbs)
In a bowl, MIX:
1 tbsp extra virgin olive oil
2 tbsp red wine vinegar
¼ tsp dried rosemary, crushed
¼ tsp dried thyme
¼ tsp dried tarragon
Dash paprika
Dash black pepper
SPRAY broiler pan with no-stick cooking spray.
PLACE breasts bone-side down and BROIL 6 inches from heat for 20 minutes.
TURN breasts up and brush with marinade. BROIL 10 minutes.
BRUSH with marinade again and BROIL about 5 minutes more.

Serves 4.

Nutritional Values per Serving

Carbohydrate	0.8 gms
Protein	58.5 gms
Calories	419
Fat	18.8 gms
Fiber	0.1 gms

Grilled Chicken Breasts With Mustard

. . . . add grapevine, mesquite chips, or hickory chips to the coals for a variety of grilled flavors. Makes an elegant summer barbecue.

WASH and PAT DRY
4 chicken breast halves (skin on)

MUSTARD MARINADE
MIX until well blended:
¼ cup Dijon mustard
¼ cup old-style mustard with seeds
¼ cup hot German mustard
¼ cup white wine vinegar
¼ cup extra virgin olive oil
4 packets Equal or Sweet'N Low
juice of ½ lemon
1 shallot sliced (or substitute ½ onion)
coarsely ground black pepper

MARINATE chicken breasts at least 3 hours before grilling.
GRILL over medium-hot to red-hot coals for 6 to 7 minutes per
    side.
Lightly WARM some of the remaining marinade to serve as a
    sauce over the chicken.

Serves 4.

Nutritional Values per Serving

Carbohydrate	1.7 gms
Protein	30.4 gms
Calories	290
Fat	17.9 gms
Fiber	0.0 gms

Roman-Style Chicken

. . . . this chicken dish, created by Bill Parker, will be one you will want to serve over and over again. Never has plain old chicken tasted this good!

WASH and SEASON   *6 large chicken breasts or thighs*
SET ASIDE.
CHOP   *1 onion*
SAUTÉ it in   *2 tbsp butter and 2 tbsp olive oil*
ADD the chicken and CONTINUE COOKING until chicken
    browns slightly.
ADD   *1 14½-oz can tomatoes (chopped) and*
          their juice
          ½ tsp garlic powder
          1 tbsp sweet basil
          ½ tsp oregano
COVER and SIMMER for 20 minutes.

Meanwhile:
CLEAN and CUT   *1 bell pepper into medium strips*
WASH and SLICE   *½ lb fresh mushrooms*
          4 medium zucchini squash

In a second pan:
SAUTÉ bell pepper in   *2 tbsp butter and 2 tbsp olive oil*
          until soft.
ADD mushrooms and zucchini. SAUTÉ until mushrooms shrink
    and absorb butter and oil.
ADD this mixture to the chicken.
COVER again and SIMMER another 20 minutes.
REMOVE from heat.
STIR IN   *¼ cup grated parmesan cheese*

Serves 6.

Nutritional Values per Serving

Carbohydrate	8 gms
Protein	30 gms
Calories	313
Fat	17 gms
Fiber	2 gms

Roasted Paprika Chicken

. . . . just when you thought there was no other way to make chicken, here comes a spicy alternative.

WASH and DRAIN   *1 whole roasting hen*

BRUSH   *1–2 tbsp olive oil onto chicken*

RUB   *2 tsp salt and pepper onto chicken and into cavity*

PEEL AND QUARTER   *1 whole onion, place into cavity*

SPRINKLE   *liberally with paprika*

PLACE in roasting pan SPRAYED first with no-stick cooking spray.

COVER with foil while BAKING 45 minutes at 400°.

UNCOVER and BAKE another 15 minutes until skin is crisp.

Serves 4.

Nutritional Values per Serving

Carbohydrate   0.9 gms
Protein   39.0 gms
Calories   278
Fat   12.5 gms
Fiber   0.0 gms

Barbecued Chicken Wings

. . . . this recipe, developed by Bill Parker, is perfect for a big celebration in the summertime, a Fourth of July cookout, a picnic, or in smaller quantities just for dinner.

Earlier in the day, make a dipping sauce as follows:
In a saucepan:

MIX TOGETHER *1 cup water*
½ cup olive oil
½ cup vinegar
2 tbsp chili powder
½ tsp cayenne pepper

BRING TO A BOIL, continue boiling 5 minutes, SET ASIDE.

CHOP TIPS from *5–6 lbs chicken wings*
SPRINKLE lightly with *salt and pepper*
COVER

BRING COALS of a covered grill to medium-hot heat.
ARRANGE wings on grill. COVER and SMOKE. TURN wings and rearrange frequently to prevent burning. COOK until the wings begin to seem a bit dry (about 1–1½ hours).
REMOVE wings from grill with tongs and immediately DIP hot wings into dipping sauce and place onto serving platter.

Serves 10–12.

Nutritional Values per Serving

Carbohydrate	1.4 gms
Protein	38.2 gms
Calories	303
Fat	16.8 gms
Fiber	0.0 gms

French Onion Chicken Breasts

. . . . this dish can be put together ahead of time and popped into the oven when you get home from a busy day. It's easy and tasty.

PREHEAT oven to 400°.
WASH and pat dry   *4 or 5 chicken breasts*
SPRINKLE with   *salt and pepper to taste*
ARRANGE in a 9 × 13 baking dish.
POUR over chicken   *1 can French onion soup (canned)*
COVER with foil.
BAKE at 400° for 30 to 35 minutes.
REMOVE foil and continue to bake another 10 minutes to brown
  skin a little.

Serves 4 or 5.

Nutritional Values per Serving

Carbohydrate	2.9 gms
Protein	58.0 gms
Calories	420
Fat	19.7 gms
Fiber	0.1 gms

Skillet Chicken Italiano

. . . . it's the same old chicken, but this time with the flavor of sun-drenched Italy. Easy and quick and delicious.

In a wok or large skillet over high heat:

HEAT	*3 tbsp olive oil*
SAUTÉ	*1 clove garlic, minced*
ADD	*2 large chicken breasts, skinned, boned, and cut into 1" cubes*
	1 cup frozen Italian green beans, thawed
	½ cup chopped red bell pepper
	½ tsp salt

STIR FRY about 3 minutes.

ADD	*2 whole tomatoes, quartered*
	4 mashed anchovies (made to a paste)
	2 tbsp diced pimento
	1 tbsp capers, rinsed and drained

STIR FRY about 1 minute.

SPRINKLE with *1 to 2 tbsp fresh lemon juice*

TURN onto platter and SERVE.

Serves 4.

Nutritional Values per Serving

Carbohydrate	6.6 gms
Protein	31.6 gms
Calories	320
Fat	18.4 gms
Fiber	1.7 gms

Chicken Tabasco

. . . . around our house, the kids will lay odds that the main course at dinner will be chicken. Since we have a multitude of hungry boys to feed, we eat a lot of it. This recipe is another of our favorites that can be put together beforehand (we often do it the night before) and popped into the oven an hour before dinner.

PREHEAT oven to 350°.
WASH and dry   *1 3-lb chicken, cut up*
COMBINE   *1 tsp Krazy Mixed-up Salt*
                      ¼ tsp Tabasco sauce
                      ½ tsp paprika
                      2 tbsp lime juice
                      2 tbsp olive oil

PLACE chicken in a baking dish. POUR Tabasco mixture over chicken.

MARINATE in refrigerator at least 2 hours. BRING to room temperature before cooking.

BAKE at 350° for 1 hour, TURNING once, BASTING every 10 minutes.

Serves 6.

Nutritional Values per Serving

Carbohydrate	0.2 gms
Protein	39.0 gms
Calories	278
Fat	12.5 gms
Fiber	0.0 gms

Chicken Divan

. . . . the classic chicken dish using the versatile crème fraîche. Our young-est son will sometimes ask if he has to eat the green stuff, but what's new? The answer is, of course, yes!

PREHEAT oven to 350°.
STEAM until crisp/tender
1¼ lb broccoli flowerets
DRAIN and reserve juices.
SPRAY an 8″ baking dish with no-stick spray.
ARRANGE broccoli on it.
SLICE thinly and set aside
12 oz cooked chicken breast
In a saucepan:
HEAT
1⅓ cups reserved broccoli juice plus water if needed
STIR in
1 cup crème fraîche*
⅛ tsp nutmeg
⅛ tsp pepper
1½ tsp instant chicken bouillon granules
STIR until thickened.
POUR half the sauce over the broccoli. LAYER sliced chicken on
    top, POUR remaining sauce over chicken.
SPRINKLE with
¼ cup grated Parmesan cheese
Paprika to garnish
BAKE covered at 350° until bubbly, about 25 minutes.

Serves 6.

*See Appendix B for source for delicious crème fraîche.

Nutritional Values per Serving

Carbohydrate	4.8 gms
Protein	18.1 gms
Calories	200
Fat	12.2 gms
Fiber	2.2 gms

Sunday Spicy Chicken

. . . . a taste reminiscent of my granny's southern-fried variety, but lighter on the breading and baked instead.

PREHEAT oven to 375°.
BRUSH
4 pounds of chicken pieces with olive oil

In a large bowl:
COMBINE
½ cup Colonial light bread crumbs
¼ tsp thyme
½ tsp paprika
¼ tsp salt
¼ tsp marjoram
¼ tsp celery seed
¼ tsp black pepper
DREDGE chicken pieces in the coating.
ARRANGE them on a nonstick baking sheet.
BAKE at 375° for 45 minutes, until crisp on outside.

Serves 8.

Nutritional Values per Serving

Carbohydrate	1.6 gms
Protein	58.7 gms
Calories	376
Fat	14.5 gms
Fiber	0.1 gms

Cinder's Lemon Chicken

. . . . one of the first nurses we ever hired at our clinics loved to cook for a crowd, and since she lived alone, the clinic staff was often treated at lunch to a batch of Cinder's Lemon Chicken.

CUT into wedges   *2 large lemons*
WASH   *3 pounds chicken pieces*
ARRANGE pieces in a baking dish.
SPRINKLE with   *salt and pepper and the juice from the lemons*
LAY juiced lemon wedges atop chicken pieces.

In a separate bowl:
COMBINE   *1 onion, cut into chunks*
                       1 clove garlic, minced
                       1 tsp each thyme, marjoram, pepper
                       1 tbsp fresh parsley, chopped
                       ⅓ cup olive oil
POUR this mixture over the chicken pieces.
COVER and MARINATE in the refrigerator for several hours.
PREHEAT oven to 350° and allow chicken to come to room
    temperature.
BAKE, COVERED, for 1½ hours.

Serves 4—6.

Nutritional Values per Serving

Carbohydrate   3.0 gms
Protein   59.3 gms
Calories   400
Fat   15.0 gms
Fiber   1.0 gms

Stuffed Veal

. . . . . a touch of class, but virtually a no-fault recipe. Look for the veal on special at the meat market. Makes a fabulous presentation for entertaining.

PREHEAT oven to 350°.

WASH and POUND flat	*4 veal cutlets*
SEASON with	*½ tsp salt, or to taste*
TOP cutlets with	*4 slices boiled ham (one each)*
	4 slices Swiss cheese (one each)

ROLL up and TIE with string.

DIP rolls in	*1 well-beaten egg*
ROLL in	*¼ cup Parmesan cheese, grated*

MELT in a skillet   *4 tbsp butter*
SAUTÉ veal rolls until brown all around.
REMOVE to an ovenproof dish. POUR on sauce from pan.

ADD	*¼ cup dry white wine*
TOP with	*2 slices Swiss cheese*

BAKE at 350° for 30 minutes. REMOVE strings and serve.

Serves 4.

Nutritional Values per Serving

Carbohydrate	2.6 gms
Protein	42.8 gms
Calories	541
Fat	37.4 gms
Fiber	0.1 gms

French Onion Pork Chops

. . . . when the workday doesn't end until eight, and the kids greet you at the door with—"We're starving. What's for dinner?"—you'll be glad you put this recipe together ahead; in forty-five minutes the little dears will be fed.

SPRAY a 9 × 13 baking dish with no-stick cooking spray.
ARRANGE in dish
4 6-oz pork chops
Salt and pepper chops to taste and place in dish.
POUR over chops
1 can concentrated French onion soup
COVER with foil and BAKE at 400° for 1 hour.

Serves 4.

Nutritional Values per Serving

Carbohydrate	4.1 gms
Protein	48.0 gms
Calories	398
Fat	24.0 gms
Fiber	0.0 gms

Hobo Dinner Pork Chops

. . . . here's one that doesn't even mess up a dish. The kids think they're camping out, and there is no cleanup chore.

CUT 4 12″ squares of aluminum foil.
SPRAY lightly with no-stick cooking spray.
CLEAN and CUT into pieces
2 carrots
2 small zucchini squash
1 cooking onion
½ head cauliflower
PLACE in the center of each square
1 pork chop, seasoned to taste (total of 4 pork chops needed)
TOP each with
2 tbsp cream of celery soup concentrate
¼ of each kind of fresh vegetable
BRING corners of foil up to center and seal seams to make
   "tents." Store in refrigerator until cooking time.
PLACE tents on cookie sheet and BAKE at 400° for 45–50
   minutes.

Serves 4.

Nutritional Values per Serving

Carbohydrate	17.5 gms
Protein	48.0 gms
Calories	478
Fat	24.0 gms
Fiber	3.6 gms

Easy Beef or Pork Tenderloin

. . . . the easiest, moistest, most delicious recipe. Serve thicker slices for dinner or slice it very thin for a cocktail buffet, and it will be a hit.

PREHEAT oven to 500°.
SPRAY a baking dish with no-stick cooking spray.

On a piece of waxed paper:
MIX
1 tbsp salt
1 tbsp black pepper
2 tsp garlic powder
ROLL
2-lb tenderloin in spices to coat

PLACE loin in baking dish and place uncovered in hot oven.
Beef loin: Turn oven off immediately.
Pork loin: Leave oven on approximately 10 minutes, then turn
   off.

DO NOT OPEN OVEN DOOR for 4 hours or more. The residual
   heat from the oven will cook the loin to perfection without
   drying it out. Slice, serve.

Serves 6–8.

Nutritional Values per Serving

Carbohydrate	1.4 gms
Protein	22.0 gms
Calories	312
Fat	23.0 gms
Fiber	0.3 gms

Roast Pork Stir-fry

. . . . this recipe is a great way to use leftover pork tenderloin. That is, of course, if there is any leftover pork tenderloin.

CUT into 1" cubes
2 cups roasted pork
HEAT a wok or skillet.
COMBINE in skillet
the pork
2 onions, cut in chunks
2 tbsp soy sauce
2 tbsp water
COOK on high heat for 1 or 2 minutes.
ADD
1 oz unsweetened pineapple juice
¾ lb fresh asparagus, cut into 1" lengths
⅓ cup fresh mushrooms, sliced
COOK 5 or 6 minutes more.
ADD
½ cup tomato, chopped
DISSOLVE
1 tsp cornstarch or Solka Floc* in ¼ cup white wine or vinegar
STIR into meat mixture, stirring constantly for 2 or 3 minutes
     until sauce thickens and vegetables are tender.

Serves 4.

*See Appendix B for sources for Solka Floc.

Nutritional Values per Serving

Carbohydrate	12.6 gms
Protein	20.1 gms
Calories	319
Fat	21.2 gms
Fiber	2.5 gms

Weight-Loss Chili

. . . . *this recipe works well for the weight-loss phase of the diet as well as maintenance. When I make chili, I like to keep the meat coarsely ground and the vegetables chopped into good-size chunks. The fancy red kidney beans that I love to put into my chili have too great a carbohydrate count to work well during the weight-loss phase of the diet. Save them for later.*

1 pound lean ground beef
¼ cup chopped onion
¼ cup sliced or chopped mushrooms
¼ cup diced bell pepper
1 small can sliced or whole tomatoes (if whole used, cut into pieces first)
2 tbsp Mexene Chili Powder (more or less to taste)
Salt

SPRAY a skillet with no-stick cooking spray. Quickly SAUTÉ
   onion, pepper, then ADD and sauté mushrooms. Set aside.
BROWN ground beef and drain fat.
In a deep saucepan or stockpot:
COMBINE browned beef, onion, mushrooms, pepper, tomatoes,
   and enough water to achieve desired thickness.
BLEND in chili powder and salt to taste. SIMMER about 30
   minutes.

Serves 4.

Nutritional Values per Serving

Carbohydrate	6.1 gms
Protein	20.9 gms
Calories	274
Fat	18.7 gms
Fiber	0.9 gms

Mom's Meat Loaf

. . . . whose meat loaf could be better? I was probably one of the few children in the history of the world who truly loved my mother's meat loaf. I still do.

1½ *pounds lean ground beef*
½ *cup minced raw onion*
½ *cup diced bell pepper*
3 slices Colonial light white bread, toasted and cubed
1 egg
¼ *cup milk*
1 tbsp French's Worcestershire sauce
salt and pepper to taste

SPRAY skillet with no-stick cooking spray. SAUTÉ onion and green pepper. Set aside.

In large mixing bowl, BEAT egg well, ADD milk, onion, bell pepper, Worcestershire sauce and MIX well. ADD ground beef and toasted bread cubes. Thoroughly MIX ingredients and turn out into a microwave-proof loaf pan that has been sprayed with no-stick cooking spray.

MICROWAVE on full power for 15 minutes. Turn and microwave for another 10 to 12 minutes at 80% power (medium high).
OR you may BAKE in conventional oven at 350° for 1 hour.

Serves 6.

Nutritional Values per Serving

Carbohydrate	7.8 gms
Protein	22.8 gms
Calories	309
Fat	20.2 gms
Fiber	0.5 gms

Beef K-Bobs

. . . . we like to marinate the meat overnight when possible, but if pressed for time, or on the spur of the moment, a quick tenderizing in Worcestershire sauce or olive oil marinade for 15 or 20 minutes will do. Add a little grapevine or hickory to the coals for a distinctive flavor.

TENDERIZE and SEASON	*16 1" cubes of steak*
CLEAN	*16 whole fresh mushrooms*
PEEL and QUARTER	*4 small onions*
PEEL, CLEAN, and QUARTER	*4 small bell peppers*

On 4 or 5 wooden or metal skewers:
ARRANGE meat, pepper, onion, and mushroom in repeating
    pattern until the skewer is full.
BRUSH all with olive oil.
SPRINKLE with ground black pepper.
GRILL over medium- to red-hot coals for 4 minutes a side or
    until done.

Serves 4. Good with salad.

Nutritional Values per Serving

Carbohydrate	12.1 gms
Protein	19.7 gms
Calories	251.5
Fat	14.2 gms
Fiber	3.2 gms

Grilled Salmon Steaks With Chive Butter

. . . . in Little Rock, we wait in July as patiently as we can for Fresh Salmon Week at the supermarket. The remainder of the year, we can get very nice frozen salmon steaks. Good, but certainly not as delicately wonderful as the truly fresh. We save this recipe for that magic week.

4 1-inch thick (6-oz) salmon steaks
olive oil
chive butter (see below)

BRUSH salmon with olive oil. GRILL over medium-hot coals on an open grill about 5 to 6 minutes per side. PLACE a pat of chive butter onto each hot steak to serve.

Serves 4.

CHIVE BUTTER
Allow stick of butter to SOFTEN in a bowl until malleable. With a fork, BLEND in: *a dash of lemon juice*
1 tsp fresh minced parsley
1 tbsp fresh minced chives
salt and pepper to taste
FORM the butter into a 6"-long log on a sheet of waxed paper. WRAP securely and REFRIGERATE until hardened. Use as needed.
Makes about 12–15 pats of butter.

Nutritional Values per Serving

Carbohydrate	0.6 gms
Protein	27.2 gms
Calories	282
Fat	18.6 gms
Fiber	0.1 gms

Grilled or Broiled Halibut Steaks

. . . . any light-tasting, firm-fleshed fish steak will work well here. Marinating overnight enhances the flavor immeasurably.

SELECT *4 ¾-inch thick (6-oz) halibut steaks*
PLACE them into a large zip-closure bag.
ADD *¼ cup extra virgin olive oil*
  1 tsp minced garlic
  1 tsp black pepper
  1 tsp Mrs. Dash (spicy flavor)
MARINATE overnight in refrigerator, turning bag over
  occasionally.
GRILL over red-hot coals 4 minutes per side.
Or, BROIL under oven broiler 4 minutes per side.

Serves 4.

Nutritional Values per Serving

Carbohydrate	0.5 gms
Protein	22.8 gms
Calories	240
Fat	16.0 gms
Fiber	0.1 gms

Fish and Peppers

. . . . this is fish with some heat. How much depends upon how liberal you'd like to get with the chilies. Suit your taste, but the amount suggested tends toward the moderately spicy.

PREHEAT broiler.
BLEND well

1 canned green chili pepper (minced and seeded)
2 cloves minced garlic
2 tbsp lemon juice
3 tbsp softened butter
1 tbsp parsley, minced
½ tsp black pepper

WASH and pat dry
1 pound sole or flounder fillets
SPREAD pepper mixture evenly on both sides of fillets.
MARINATE for 20 minutes.
BROIL for 10 minutes, or until flaky.

Serves 4.

Nutritional Values per Serving

Carbohydrate	1.7 gms
Protein	15.5 gms
Calories	140
Fat	7.8 gms
Fiber	0.1 gms

Halibut Jardiniere

. . . . a Triple-Crown winner: low-fat, low-carbohydrate, and low-calorie. The only thing this recipe is not low on is taste. It's great!

PREHEAT oven to 350°.
SPRAY a baking dish with no-stick cooking spray.
LINE bottom of dish with
⅔ cup thin onion slices
PLACE atop onion
8 halibut steaks

In a separate bowl:
COMBINE
⅓ cup tomato, chopped
⅓ cup green pepper, chopped
¼ cup fresh parsley, chopped
3 tbsp pimento, chopped
1½ cups fresh chopped mushrooms
SPREAD mixture over fish steaks.

BLEND
⅓ cup dry white wine
2 tbsp lime juice
1 tsp salt
¼ tsp dillweed
¼ tsp black pepper
POUR over fish and vegetables.
BAKE at 350° for 25 minutes, until fish flakes with a fork.
GARNISH with lime wedges or slices.

Serves 8.

Nutritional Values per Serving

Carbohydrate	2.9 gms
Protein	20.7 gms
Calories	125
Fat	2.4 gms
Fiber	0.7 gms

Shrimp K-Bobs

. . . . we love to give our grill a workout in the summer, and k-bobs are one of the family favorites. This shrimp variety is mouth-watering and easy.

CLEAN, peel, and devein	*16 large shrimp*
CLEAN	*16 large whole fresh mushrooms*
PEEL and quarter	*4 small onions*
PEEL, clean, and quarter	*4 bell peppers*

On 4 to 5 wooden or metal skewers:
ARRANGE shrimp, pepper, onion, and mushroom in repeating pattern until skewer is full.
BRUSH all with olive oil.
SPRINKLE with pepper.
GRILL over medium- to red-hot coals for 4 minutes a side or until done.

Serves 4 or 5.

Nutritional Values per Serving

Carbohydrate	12.1 gms
Protein	26.3 gms
Calories	229
Fat	8.7 gms
Fiber	3.2 gms

Shrimp Scampi

. . . . needs no introduction, but this version is quick and delicious. Doubles or triples well for a bigger crowd.

PREHEAT broiler.
SHELL and devein   *1 lb medium shrimp*
SQUEEZE onto shrimp *1 juiced lemon*
SET ASIDE for 20 minutes.

In a separate bowl:
MIX
¼ cup Parmesan cheese, grated
1 tsp garlic powder
DIP shrimp in cheese mixture.
PLACE on broiler pan.
TOP each with   *½ slice bacon (takes about 7 slices, total)*
BROIL until shrimp are bright pink.

Serves 3.

Nutritional Values per Serving

Carbohydrate	1.7 gms
Protein	35.2 gms
Calories	255
Fat	11.2 gms
Fiber	0.0 gms

Tuna or Chicken Salad

. . . . everyone has his own favorite way to make tuna salad. Here is ours.

HARD-BOIL
2 eggs
COOL, peel, and chop them. Set aside.

In a mixing bowl:
COMBINE
1 can tuna or chicken, drained well
the chopped eggs
5 dill pickle slices, chopped
½ tsp garlic powder
2 tsp dried minced onion (rehydrated)
1½ tbsp mayonnaise (to taste)
1 tbsp Dijon-style mustard (to taste)
Nice served on two or three tomato slices, or as a sandwich.

Serves 2.

Nutritional Values per Serving

Carbohydrate	1.9 gms
Protein	33.7 gms
Calories	284
Fat	14.5 gms
Fiber	0.2 gms

Soups and Salads

Avgolemono (Greek Egg-and-Lemon Soup)

. . . . a tangy favorite, especially good before chicken dishes.

In a saucepan:
HEAT to boiling
2 10-ounce cans chicken broth, condensed
1½ cups water
REDUCE heat to very low.
BEAT
4 eggs until foamy
BEAT IN
¼ cup lemon juice
WHISKING constantly, slowly ADD a little hot broth to egg/
    lemon.
POUR the egg-and-lemon mixture into the pan of broth, COOK
    over low heat, STIRRING constantly until thickened.
POUR into serving bowls, GARNISH with lemon slices.

Serves 6–8.

Nutritional Values per Serving

Carbohydrate	1.1 gms
Protein	4.5 gms
Calories	52
Fat	3.2 gms
Fiber	0.0 gms

Homestyle Tomato Soup

. . . . *the first day that the air takes on that unmistakable crispness of fall, we break out the stockpot and treat ourselves to homemade soup. This low-carbohydrate version comes from Bill Parker of Memphis, but it doesn't take a master chef to prepare it.*

In a large saucepan:

HEAT	*⅛ cup olive oil*
SAUTÉ	*1 medium onion, thinly sliced*
	2 large cloves garlic, crushed
	1 14½-oz can whole tomatoes, chopped
ADD	*3 cans beef bouillon or broth*
	¼ cup chopped parsley (fresh if possible)
	½ tsp black pepper
	1 tsp basil

SIMMER for 30 minutes.

Serves 4.

Nutritional Values per Serving

Carbohydrates	8.8 gms
Protein	4.4 gms
Calories	115
Fat	6.7 gms
Fiber	1.5 gms

Sadie Kendall's Mushroom Soup

. . . . this is the richest, most elegant cream of mushroom soup I have ever tasted. And it doesn't take hours of slaving over a hot stove. Delicious as a first course or as lunch with a sandwich or salad.

In a heavy saucepan:

MELT	*1 tbsp unsalted butter*
SAUTÉ	*2 tbsp minced shallots (or onion)*
ADD	*1 lb fresh, firm mushrooms, chopped coarsely*
	¼ tsp dried thyme
	½ bay leaf

SAUTÉ until mushrooms release their liquid.

ADD	*1 tsp salt*
	½ tsp fresh-ground black pepper
	1½ cups chicken stock

SIMMER for 10 minutes.

ADD   *1 cup crème fraîche**

SIMMER 2 minutes more.

ADJUST seasonings and serve warm.

Serves 4.

*See Appendix B for source of crème fraîche.

Nutritional Values per Serving

Carbohydrate	5.7 gms
Protein	4.7 gms
Calories	179.5
Fat	15.8 gms
Fiber	0.7 gms

Butter Lettuce Salad

. . . . an elegant offering when company comes and a welcome change from a tossed salad.

WASH, dry, and tear
1 medium head butter lettuce
CHILL in a cotton kitchen towel for several hours in refrigerator.
In a small bowl:
MIX together   *¼ cup olive or walnut oil*
                     1 tbsp wine vinegar
                     1 packet Equal or Sweet'N Low
                     ½ tsp each salt and ground pepper
At serving time:
PLACE chilled greens into salad bowl.
ADD   *1 small can mandarin orange slices in water, drained*
                     ½ cup large walnut pieces
TOSS with dressing (above) to coat well.

Serves 3 to 4.

Nutritional Values per Serving

Carbohydrate	5.7 gms
Protein	4.5 gms
Calories	231
Fat	22.5 gms
Fiber	2.5 gms

Chef's Salad

. . . . *a luncheon favorite. This salad works well for using up whatever you have on hand. Just toss in the leftover chicken, beef, pork roast, or shrimp in place of the ham.*

WASH and TEAR *1 cup iceberg lettuce*
               1 cup loose leaf lettuce
ADD   *1 hard-boiled egg, sliced*
               ¼ cup shredded carrots
               ¼ cup chopped green onion
               ⅓ cucumber, peeled and sliced
               ½ tomato, cut in wedges
               1 oz diced or julienne ham
               1 oz shredded hard cheese
TOP with your favorite low-carbohydrate dressing and fresh-ground pepper.

Serves 1.

Nutritional Values per Serving

Carbohydrate	11.7 gms
Protein	21.1 gms
Calories	272
Fat	16.0 gms
Fiber	4.0 gms

Vegetable Dishes

Asparagus Jayme

. . . . Jayme, a dear friend of ours, brought this dish already prepared to the house one evening for supper. I have loved asparagus for as long as I can remember, but this simple rendition is now my personal favorite.

8 nice stalks of fresh asparagus
2 tbsp extra virgin olive oil
1 clove garlic, crushed
2 tsps white wine vinegar

BRING water to boil in a shallow pan or skillet.
WASH and TRIM ends from asparagus.
PLACE asparagus in boiling water just until it turns a bright green color. REMOVE promptly and SUBMERGE in cold water to stop the cooking process. CHILL.
MIX together the olive oil and garlic and vinegar. (It is best if done ahead and left to sit for several hours to allow garlic to flavor the oil and vinegar.)
Before serving, POUR the vinegar and oil over the chilled asparagus.

Serves 2 (4 stalks each).
The recipe doubles and triples well.

Nutritional Values per Serving

Carbohydrate	2.6 gms
Protein	1.6 gms
Calories	135
Fat	13.7 gms
Fiber	0.0 gms

Sliced Fresh Tomatoes Italiano

. . . . makes a colorful addition as a side dish or a salad course.

3 ripe red tomatoes
2 tbsp tiny fresh basil leaves
⅓ cup extra virgin olive oil
salt and freshly ground black pepper to taste

WASH tomatoes and basil. SLICE tomatoes ¼ inch thick and
     ARRANGE on platter. SPRINKLE basil leaves over slices.
     POUR olive oil over tomatoes and allow to stand 30 minutes.
     SEASON to taste with salt and pepper.

Serves 4.

Nutritional Values per Serving

Carbohydrate	5.6 gms
Protein	1.1 gms
Calories	184
Fat	3.0 gms
Fiber	1.7 gms

Salad de Florette

. . . . tossed, this makes a great salad. Serve the dressing on the side, and you have a fresh veggie dip for parties.

WASH and BREAK flowerets from:
2 cups cauliflower
2 cups broccoli
PLACE into large bowl and set aside.
In a blender or processor:
BLEND until smooth
¾ cup buttermilk
½ cup cottage cheese
1½ tsp dried dillweed
½ tsp black pepper
1 tsp soy sauce
POUR dressing over flowerets and toss well.

Serves 4–6.

Nutritional Values per Serving

Carbohydrate	7.2 gms
Protein	6.3 gms
Calories	52
Fat	0.6 gms
Fiber	1.3 gms

Matilda's Marinated Green Beans

. . . . Matilda served this delightful dish at an elegant buffet at her home. We loved it. This recipe does as well at a potluck supper as at a cocktail buffet. Give the flavors time to blend well. It's delicious.

In a mixing bowl:
COMBINE
1 large can french-cut green beans
1 can water chestnuts, chopped
1 can chow mein vegetables
1 can sliced mushrooms
1 jar pimento, chopped
STIR together in a separate bowl:
⅓ cup extra virgin olive oil
¼ cup wine vinegar
6 packets Equal or Sweet'N Low sweetener
1 tsp each: salt, pepper, garlic powder
POUR marinade over vegetables, STIR to coat well, COVER and
REFRIGERATE for at least one hour to allow flavors to
combine.
SERVE cold.

Serves 4–6.

Nutritional Values per Serving

Carbohydrate	3.9 gms
Protein	0.8 gms
Calories	80
Fat	7.3 gms
Fiber	0.8 gms

Grilled Zucchini

. . . . great with steaks, chops, chicken, or fish. A side dish on the grill in the summer when it's too hot to turn on the oven.

CLEAN and TRIM ends from
4 large zucchini
SLICE approximately ¼" thick, lengthwise.
BRUSH both sides of cut zucchini with olive oil.
SPRINKLE on a dash of salt, pepper, garlic powder, and
    Parmesan cheese.
GRILL over medium-hot coals for 10 minutes, turning frequently,
    or
BROIL under oven broiler for 4–5 minutes per side.

Serves 4–6.

Nutritional Values per Serving

Carbohydrate	4.6 gms
Protein	2.0 gms
Calories	87
Fat	7.4 gms
Fiber	1.8 gms

Fancy Green Beans

. . . . these look elegant enough for company, but they are easy enough for everyday.

WASH and TRIM ends from   *1 lb fresh green beans*
STEAM beans about 7–8 minutes (until they turn bright green).
In a skillet:
MELT   *2 tbsp butter*
ADD and sauté   *steamed beans*
                          1 small can sliced water chestnuts
SEASON with salt and pepper.

Serves 4–6.

Nutritional Values per Serving

Carbohydrate	4.6 gms
Protein	0.9 gms
Calories	56
Fat	4.1 gms
Fiber	0.8 gms

Italian Zucchini Bake

. . . . a side dish with an opulent flair that tastes expensive, but isn't.

WASH and CUT into rounds
4 large zucchini
In a skillet:
MELT   *2 tbsp butter*
ADD   *1 clove minced garlic*
                        1 onion, chopped
SAUTÉ until transparent.
ADD the zucchini and sauté about 5 minutes, until tender.
PEEL and CHOP   *2 small tomatoes*
ADD to tomatoes *2 tbsp snipped fresh parsley*
SPRAY a baking dish with no-stick cooking spray.
LAYER tomatoes, then zucchini, then
                ⅛ cup shredded cheddar cheese.
REPEAT the layers and sprinkle top with black pepper.
BAKE at 350°F for 40 minutes.

Serves 6.

Nutritional Values per Serving

Carbohydrate	7.0 gms
Protein	3.4 gms
Calories	95
Fat	6.7 gms
Fiber	2.4 gms

Tangy Cabbage

. . . . a traditional favorite from the South, where we know how to panfry everything from pickles to peaches.

SHRED
2 cups cabbage
In a saucepan:
MELT
1 tbsp butter
ADD
cabbage
and STIR to coat with butter
¼ cup water
½ tsp salt
STIR and COVER to SIMMER for 10 minutes.
DRAIN cabbage and set aside.
In the saucepan on burner:
COMBINE
1 tbsp white vinegar
2 packets Equal or Sweet'N Low
½ tsp Dijon-style mustard
COVER and SIMMER on very low heat for 1 minute.
In a bowl:
COMBINE
2 tbsp sour cream
2 tbsp mayonnaise
ADD the mustard sauce and FOLD this mixture into cabbage.
STIR well to coat.

Serves 2.

Nutritional Values per Serving

Carbohydrate	6.3 gms
Protein	1.9 gms
Calories	208
Fat	20.3 gms
Fiber	1.8 gms

Cukes and Onions

. . . . this light side dish or salad does well made ahead, made in double or triple quantity, and is even great as a snack.

PEEL and SLICE very thin
2 cucumbers
2 white onions
PLACE into a bowl.
SPRINKLE with
1 tsp salt
TOSS, COVER, and set aside for 1 hour.
DRAIN off liquid.
In a separate bowl:
COMBINE
2 tbsp white vinegar
¼ cup water
1 packet Equal or Sweet'N Low
POUR vinegar mixture over cucumbers and onions and
   REFRIGERATE for several hours. Can be prepared up to 24
   hours in advance.

Serves 4–6.

Nutritional Values per Serving

Carbohydrate	5.2 gms
Protein	0.8 gms
Calories	23
Fat	0.2 gms
Fiber	1.4 gms

Zucchini Medley

. . . . chop and slice the vegetables ahead, and this side dish can be ready in just a few minutes.

In a large skillet:
MELT
2 tbsp butter
SAUTÉ
1 tsp minced garlic until transparent
ADD
1 large fresh tomato, diced
1 tsp fresh parsley, chopped fine
½ tsp oregano
½ tsp coarsely ground black pepper
½ cup water
COOK over medium-high heat for 3 minutes.
Meanwhile:
STEAM until crisp
2 large zucchini, sliced in rounds
1½ cups cauliflowerets
ADD the vegetables to the skillet and COOK, STIRRING, 5
   minutes more.
SPRINKLE on
2 tbsp Parmesan or Romano cheese

Serves 5–6.

Nutritional Values per Serving

Carbohydrate	4.0 gms
Protein	2.1 gms
Calories	52
Fat	3.5 gms
Fiber	1.5 gms

Skillet Ratatouille

. . . . serve this dish on the side for six or eight, or as a main dish for four. Either way it's a winner, especially in the summer when the vegetables are at their peak of freshness.

CLEAN, PEEL, and coarsely CHOP
1 large eggplant
4 medium zucchini
1 large white onion
3 cloves garlic
1 large bell pepper
2 large tomatoes
2 tbsp chopped parsley
In a skillet:
HEAT
2 tbsp olive oil
SAUTÉ
onion and garlic until transparent
Then ADD
eggplant, zucchini, bell pepper, tomatoes, and parsley
SEASON with
1 tsp dried oregano
1 tsp dried basil
salt and pepper to taste
Continue to SAUTÉ, STIRRING to prevent sticking, until
    vegetables are tender.

Serves 4.

Nutritional Values per Serving

Carbohydrate	15.4 gms
Protein	3.2 gms
Calories	129
Fat	7.4 gms
Fiber	5.1 gms

Seasoned Green Beans

. . . . no matter how you slice them, green beans are a bargain for the low-carbohydrate dieter. This variation on the old favorite comes to us courtesy of Bill Parker of Memphis, Tennessee. We've always known Bill was a great cook, but the ease and delectable taste of this simple dish prove it.

In a saucepan:
DRAIN juice from
1 can whole or french-cut green beans
COMBINE
juice from beans
⅛ tsp tarragon
½ tsp basil
½ tsp dried parsley
¼ tsp dried fennel (crushed)
¼ stick butter
SIMMER about 10 minutes. REMOVE from heat. ADD beans and
    STIR well to coat. SERVE with a dollop of sour cream.

Serves 2.

Nutritional Values per Serving

Carbohydrate	4.9 gms
Protein	1.7 gms
Calories	150
Fat	15.0 gms
Fiber	1.1 gms

Easy Marinated Brussels Sprouts

. . . . an interesting side dish, and the perfect dish for stand-up cocktail buffets. Tangy and different.

According to package directions:
COOK
about 2 cups frozen brussels sprouts
DRAIN.
ADD
1 cup Newman's Own Au Naturel Vinaigrette salad dressing
COVER and REFRIGERATE at least overnight.
SERVE cold or REWARM for a few minutes.

Serves 4 as a side dish. Great on toothpicks at parties.

Nutritional Values per Serving

Carbohydrate	7.3 gms
Protein	2.8 gms
Calories	176
Fat	16.3 gms
Fiber	2.3 gms

Sautéed Broccoli

. . . . the perfect low-carbohydrate vegetable just got better. Low in carbohydrates and calories, high in fiber and potassium, and absolutely delicious.

In a large skillet:
HEAT   *4 tsp olive oil*
SAUTÉ   *2 cloves garlic, chopped*
ADD   *1 10-oz pkg frozen broccoli, thawed*
COOK about one minute, stirring occasionally.
ADD   *½ cup chicken broth*
           1 tbsp fresh lemon juice
           ¼ tsp grated lemon peel
           ¼ tsp pepper
REDUCE heat. COVER and SIMMER for 5–7 minutes, until
   broccoli is crisp-tender.

Serves 4.

Nutritional Values per Serving

Carbohydrate	4.1 gms
Protein	2.5 gms
Calories	64
Fat	4.8 gms
Fiber	2.3 gms

Wilted Leaf Lettuce or Spinach Salad

. . . . at family gatherings around my parents' house, a throng usually gathers around my mother, plaintively begging her to make wilted lettuce for supper. No one can make this quintessential Southern delicacy quite like Mom, but here's the recipe. Give it a try. If you've never had this dish, you're in for an incredible surprise.

COOK and CRUMBLE   6 pieces bacon
To the bacon drippings in the skillet:
ADD   ¼ cup vinegar
                         2 packets Equal or Sweet'N Low
                         ¼ cup water
STIR and BRING to a boil.

In a large salad bowl:
COMBINE   8 cups torn leaf lettuce or spinach
                         ½ cup chopped green onions
                         6 radishes, thinly sliced
ADD the crumbled bacon. POUR on the hot dressing and TOSS to coat and wilt slightly. Garnish with chopped hard-boiled egg if desired. Serve immediately.

Serves 6 to 8.

Nutritional Values per Serving

Carbohydrate	3.0 gms
Protein	2.8 gms
Calories	45
Fat	2.3 gms
Fiber	1.0 gms

Herbed Brussels Sprouts

. . . . my wife's mother told her these vegetables were "baby cabbages" when she was a kid. Only then would she eat them. Times change, palates change, and these sprouts taste great.

STEAM about 10 minutes   *10 oz frozen brussels sprouts*
                                      1 small onion, thinly sliced

In a saucepan:
MELT   *1 tbsp butter*
SAUTÉ until brown   *1 clove garlic, minced*
ADD   *the steamed sprouts and onion*
                                        ¼ tsp thyme
                                        ¼ tsp oregano
                                        ¼ tsp salt
                                        ¼ tsp pepper
COOK, stirring occasionally, for 4 to 5 minutes, until vegetables are heated through.

Serves 4.

Nutritional Values per Serving

Carbohydrate	7.4 gms
Protein	2.4 gms
Calories	63
Fat	3.4 gms
Fiber	2.1 gms

Sassy Green Beans

. . . . there is a definite Italian flair to these beans.

WASH and CUT to 1"   *¾ lb whole fresh green beans*
In a saucepan:
COMBINE   *the beans*
                             3 oz tomato juice
                             3 oz water
                             2 tbsp chopped onion
                             1 tsp oregano
                             ½ tsp basil
                             ¼ tsp garlic powder
                             ¼ tsp each salt and pepper
COVER, REDUCE HEAT, and SIMMER for 5 minutes. UNCOVER
    and COOK until green beans are tender.
SPRINKLE with   *1 tbsp Romano cheese, grated*

Serves 3 or 4.

Nutritional Values per Serving

Carbohydrate	5.7 gms
Protein	2.4 gms
Calories	38
Fat	1.2 gms
Fiber	1.2 gms

Eggplant Milano

. . . . the maligned and misunderstood eggplant serves as the basis for this side dish. Great with veal, beef, chicken, or shrimp entrées.

In a skillet:
HEAT   *2 tbsp olive oil*
ADD   *1 eggplant, peeled and coarsely chopped*
         ½ cup thickly sliced celery
         1 onion, coarsely chopped
COOK over medium heat until onion is transparent.
ADD   *2 cups tomato, coarsely chopped*
         ¼ cup red wine vinegar
         1 tsp oregano
         ¼ tsp each basil, salt, and pepper
COVER and SIMMER for 25 minutes.

Serves 6.

Nutritional Values per Serving

Carbohydrate	6.4 gms
Protein	1.0 gms
Calories	67
Fat	4.0 gms
Fiber	2.1 gms

Asparagus Parmesano

. . . . my favorite vegetable, but this time presented with a hot cheese sauce to dress it up.

WASH and TRIM ends from
1 lb fresh asparagus

In a skillet:
BRING to a boil   *water to cover asparagus*
COOK asparagus in boiling water until just bright green and
    crisp. DRAIN, REMOVE to serving dish and KEEP HOT.

In a saucepan:
MELT   *1 tbsp butter*
STIR in   *1 tbsp flour*
ADD gradually   *¼ cup chicken broth*
                  ¼ cup milk
COOK, stirring, until mixture thickens.
STIR in   *2 tbsp cheddar cheese, shredded*
                  2 tbsp grated Parmesan cheese
                  ¼ tsp each salt and pepper
POUR cheese sauce over asparagus.
SPRINKLE with   *1 more tbsp Parmesan cheese*

Serves 4.

Nutritional Values per Serving

Carbohydrate	4.8 gms
Protein	5.7 gms
Calories	92
Fat	6.3 gms
Fiber	1.1 gms

Condiments

Italian Dressing

. . . . this dressing recipe, contributed by Bill Parker, is the tangiest we've ever tried. You'll need a mortar and pestle to crush the spices, but its creator tells us that no self-respecting cook should be without one. One taste and you'll want to say, "Paul Newman, eat your heart out."

With a mortar and pestle:

PULVERIZE	*1 tsp rosemary leaves with ½ tsp salt*
ADD and PULVERIZE	*1 tsp garlic powder*
	1 tsp ground oregano
	1 tsp basil leaves
	3 red and 3 black peppercorns
	¼ tsp dillweed (or less if you're not fond of dill)
ADD spices to	*⅓ cup wine vinegar*
LET STAND for 30 minutes.	
ADD	*⅔ cup olive oil*
	juice of one lemon

MIX WELL and store in cruet or jar. Flavor is fullest if you do not refrigerate. The recipe doubles well.

MAKES about 8 ounces. Serving size 1 ounce.

Nutritional Values per Serving

Carbohydrate	1.6 gms
Protein	0.1 gms
Calories	163
Fat	18.0 gms
Fiber	0.0 gms

Tangy French Dressing

. . . . this dressing has plenty of zest. Even our kids love it.

In a blender or shaker jar with a tight-fitting lid:
COMBINE
3 tsp Krazy Mixed-Up Salt or seasoned salt
½ tsp dry mustard
1 packet Equal or Sweet'N Low
1 tsp Dijon-style mustard
1½ tsp lemon juice
1 tsp garlic powder
¼ tsp dried tarragon
5 tbsp olive oil
5 tbsp safflower or canola oil
1 raw egg—well beaten*
½ cup heavy cream
SHAKE or BLEND until well blended. CHILL 1 hour to blend
    flavors. STORE in a jar or cruet with a tight-fitting lid.

MAKES 15 servings of 1 ounce each.

Nutritional Values per Serving

Carbohydrate	0.8 gms
Protein	0.6 gms
Calories	129
Fat	14.0 gms
Fiber	0.0 gms

*A note of caution: In recipes calling for raw eggs, the eggs in their shells should be immersed in boiling water for 30 seconds prior to their use.

Roquefort Dressing

. . . . everyone doesn't have the palate for blue cheese, but for those among you who do, this low-carbohydrate variation will become one of your staples.

In a blender:
COMBINE   *½ cup sour cream*
              2 tbsp wine vinegar
              ¼ tsp tarragon
              1 packet Equal or Sweet'N Low
              1 tsp Krazy Mixed-Up Salt or season salt
              ½ tsp celery seed
              1 oz crumbled Roquefort cheese
BLEND well until dressing is smooth in consistency.
CAREFULLY FOLD IN *1 oz more crumbled Roquefort cheese*
STORE in a container with a tight-fitting lid.

Makes 7 servings of 1 ounce each.

Nutritional Values per Serving

Carbohydrate	1.2 gms
Protein	2.3 gms
Calories	66
Fat	6.0 gms
Fiber	0.0 gms

Blender Hollandaise Sauce

. . . . great over many cooked vegetables or for eggs Benedict. We have often made this hollandaise on a moment's notice to serve over steamed asparagus.

In a small saucepan:
MELT   *1 stick unsalted butter*
Meanwhile, in a blender:
BLEND   *3 egg yolks (reserve whites for another use, if desired)*
        2 tbsp fresh lemon juice
        1 dash cayenne pepper
With blender running:
ADD the melted butter in a slow stream
The sauce should thicken as you BLEND another 30 or 45
    seconds.
SERVE immediately.

Serves 4–6.

Nutritional Values per Serving

Carbohydrate   0.5 gms
Protein   1.4 gms
Calories   177
Fat   19.1 gms
Fiber   0.0 gms

Homemade Mayonnaise*

. . . . *in our kitchen, we use this simple homemade variety in preference to commercial products, not just for taste, but for the added value of the monounsaturated fatty acids in olive and canola oils. Making your own mayo may sound daunting, but believe me, it's a snap in the blender.*

In a blender:

BLEND together on high	*1 whole raw egg*†
	1 tsp dry mustard
	1 tsp salt
	1 dash cayenne pepper
	1 packet Equal or Sweet'N Low
	¼ cup olive oil

With blender running:

ADD in a *very* slow stream	*½ cup Puritan brand canola oil*
and then	*3 tbsp lemon juice*
and then *very slowly*	*¼ to ½ cup canola oil*

STOP blender to STIR DOWN if necessary.

STORE in a jar with a tight-fitting lid.

NOTE: You may wish to use all olive oil, but the taste is quite pronounced. Canola oil makes a much lighter flavor, but it requires a lesser amount of oil in the final addition, and the stream must be *very slow* and steady to prevent separation.

MAKES about 1 cup (or 16 1-tbsp servings).

Nutritional Values per Serving

Carbohydrate	0.2 gms
Protein	0.4 gms
Calories	126.2
Fat	11.0 gms
Fiber	0.0 gms

---

*I recently discovered a delicious mayonnaise made commercially by Spectrum Marketing in Petaluma, California. This product is made with canola oil and is, therefore, high in monounsaturated fat. You may use this product in any recipe calling for mayonnaise, and you should be able to find it in most health food stores. See Appendix B for further information.
†A note of caution: In recipes calling for raw eggs, the eggs in their shells should be immersed in boiling water for 30 seconds prior to their use.

Dry Rub for Meats

. . . . this rub will make you the barbecue whiz of the neighborhood.

In a zip closure bag:
COMBINE   *½ cup black pepper*
            ½ cup paprika
            ½ cup brown sugar
            1 tbsp garlic powder
            1 tbsp onion powder
            1 tbsp cayenne pepper
STORE dry rub in an airtight zip bag or jar.
USE by rubbing in a few tablespoons to season barbecued meats.
Excellent on ribs, brisket, pork roasts, chicken.
The recipe makes enough for many barbecues.

Nutritional Values per Serving

Carbohydrate	2.5 gms
Protein	0.1 gms
Calories	10
Fat	0.1 gms
Fiber	0.1 gms

Versatile Meat Marinade

. . . . in the summer, because we grill out nearly every day, I have thought we might save some time if we made this marinade ahead in fifty-five-gallon drums. The flavors blend well if you allow them to combine at least overnight in the refrigerator.

In a zip closure bag or jar . . .

MIX   *½ cup extra virgin olive oil*
             1 tsp minced garlic
             1 tsp black pepper
             1 tsp Original Herb or Cavender's Seasoning

If using for chops, steak, chicken breasts, or thick fish fillets, you may place frozen pieces directly into the zip-closure bag and defrost while marinating in the refrigerator overnight.

If cooking and marinating the same day, you will want to allow at least an hour or so at room temperature to impart flavor to the meat before grilling or baking.

Nutritional Values per Serving

Carbohydrate	4.0 gms
Protein	2.1 gms
Calories	87
Fat	3.5 gms
Fiber	1.5 gms

Mr. Ron's Barbecue Sauce

. . . . this delicious sauce is the carbohydrate-reduced version of the tangy barbecue sauce that made Ron Smith, one of my successful weight-loss patients, famous with his neighbors for whom he makes it.

In a large heavy stockpot:
COMBINE
42 oz Dia-Mel or Featherweight Diet Catsup (1 gm carbohydrate per tbsp)
32 oz white vinegar
10-oz can tomato puree
1 medium white onion, chopped
6 tbsp salt
6 tbsp black pepper
6 tbsp chili powder
6 tbsp Sweet'N Low or Sprinkle Sweet artificial sweetener
SIMMER all ingredients for 4 to 6 hours.
POUR into sterilized canning jars and seal while hot.

MAKES 84 1-ounce servings.

Nutritional Values per Serving

Carbohydrate	2.8 gms
Protein	0.3 gms
Calories	11
Fat	0.1 gms
Fiber	0.2 gms

Desserts and Preserves

Sinfully Rich Fudge

. . . . we served this ultrarich treat to guests once at a cocktail buffet, and one of our friends dubbed it the best fudge he'd ever eaten. High praise for a dessert so low in carbohydrate.

In a saucepan over low heat:

COMBINE   *1 pkg instant chocolate sugar-free pudding*
                  ½ cup heavy cream

ADD   *3 heaping tbsp crunchy peanut butter*
                  1 tbsp crème de cacao if desired

STIR until well combined and peanut butter has melted.

In the top of an old double boiler:

MELT   *1 oz Gulf Wax canning paraffin*

SLOWLY POUR melted paraffin into fudge mixture, BEATING with a mixer on medium speed until well blended.

POUR into 8 × 8 baking dish sprayed with cooking spray.

COVER with plastic wrap.

REFRIGERATE until firm. CUT into approximately 25 squares. Serve.

Serving size—1 square.

Nutritional Values per Serving

Carbohydrate	1.7 gms
Protein	1.4 gms
Calories	50
Fat	4.2 gms
Fiber	0.2 gms

Chocolate Butter Wafers

. . . . another Bill Parker special, this one really hits the spot for choca-holics.

In a mixing bowl:
SOFTEN   *1 stick butter*
ADD and MIX WELL   *⅓ cup cocoa*
                            ½ cup instant nonfat dry milk powder
Lay out 36" waxed paper on counter.

In the top of a double boiler:
MELT   *1 oz Gulf Wax canning paraffin*
ADD   *butter, milk, and cocoa mixture*
Begin to WHISK constantly with a wire whisk as mixture
    dissolves.
When totally blended, REMOVE FROM HEAT.
ADD   *1 tsp vanilla*
                            14 packets Equal or Sweet'N Low
BLEND WELL with wire whisk.
DROP by spoonfuls onto waxed paper. STIR mixture a bit after
    each spoonful.
ALLOW TO COOL for 30 minutes.
PLACE on platter lined with waxed paper, separating layers with
    more waxed paper. REFRIGERATE.

Makes about 20 pieces.

<u>Nutritional Values per Serving</u>
<u>(based on 1 piece per serving):</u>

Carbohydrate	1.0 gms
Protein	0.6 gms
Calories	52
Fat	5.3 gms
Fiber	0.0 gms

Hot Chocolate

. . . . on a chilly fall or winter evening, what could hit the spot better than a steaming mug of hot chocolate? Probably nothing, so enjoy!

In a cup or mug:

PLACE	*1 tsp baking cocoa*
	1 packet Equal or Sweet'N Low
	Dash salt or NoSalt
	Dash cinnamon
ADD	*5 oz boiling water*
	½ oz half-and-half
TOP with	*whipped heavy cream sweetened with Equal or Sweet'N Low*

Serves 1.

Nutritional Values per Serving

Carbohydrate	3.3 gms
Protein	1.2 gms
Calories	76
Fat	7.4 gms
Fiber	0.0 gms

Meringue Tart Shells

. . . . these elegant little company dessert jewels can be filled with any number of sugar-free puddings or low-carbohydrate berries and cream. It may take you a few trial runs to get them crispy. Don't open the oven door too soon.

PREHEAT oven to 250°.
In a bowl:
COMBINE   *3 egg whites*
                ¼ tsp salt
                3 packets Equal or Canadian Sucaryl
                1 tsp almond extract
BEAT until stiff.
FOLD in   *½ cup grated almonds*
                ½ cup shredded unsweetened coconut,
                if desired
DROP by *large* spoonfuls onto buttered cookie sheet.
CREATE a depression in each mound with the bottom of a glass.
BAKE for 30 minutes, then TURN OFF heat, but LEAVE oven
     door closed for another 30 minutes.
FILL with any no-bake, sugar-free filling or fruit and cream.

Serves 6.

Nutritional Values per Serving

Carbohydrate	3.1 gms
Protein	3.8 gms
Calories	33
Fat	0.5 gms
Fiber	1.7 gms

Simple Nut Crust for Desserts

. . . . this crust is exceedingly rich. Reserve it for special occasions—a little goes a long way—but enjoy it!

PREHEAT oven to 375°.

In a bowl:
COMBINE   *1¼ cups pecans or walnuts, ground*
                         4 packets Equal or Canadian Sucaryl
                         2 tbsp flour
                         ⅛ tsp salt
                         2 tbsp melted butter
CHILL for 30 minutes.
PRESS mixture into an 8-inch pie plate.
BAKE for 10 minutes.
COOL and FILL.
(If you used Equal to sweeten, fill only with no-bake fillings, as more than 10 minutes in the oven may cause it to lose its sweetness.)

MAKES one 8-inch crust (8 servings).

Nutritional Values per Serving

Carbohydrate	3.8 gms
Protein	1.4 gms
Calories	139
Fat	13.0 gms
Fiber	1.3 gms

Strawberry Cheesecake

. . . . you will wonder what you could possibly be missing on your maintenance plan with this luscious treat available to you.

PREHEAT oven to 350°.

In a blender or processor:
COMBINE   *8 oz cream cheese*
                 4 oz half-and-half
                 3 packets Sweet'N Low or Canadian Sucaryl
                 2 eggs
                 2 tsp vanilla extract
BLEND until completely smooth.
POUR into an 8-inch ceramic or Pyrex pie pan.
BAKE for 25 minutes.
CHILL well.
GARNISH with   *1 cup sliced strawberries*
                 ½ cup sour cream to which
                 1 packet Equal or Sweet'N Low is added.

Serves 6–8.

Nutritional Values per Serving

Carbohydrate   3.4 gms
Protein   4.0 gms
Calories   159
Fat   14.6 gms
Fiber   0.4 gms

Elegant Kahlua Parfait

. . . . this quick delight will have your family or guests busily guessing what the secret ingredient is. We have never served this dessert without many compliments. Rich and delicious.

COMBINE   *1 pkg instant sugar-free vanilla pudding mix*
1¾ cups milk
2 oz Kahlua Liqueur (the ''secret'')
MIX WELL and pour into 4 parfait or dessert glasses. Set aside.

At serving time:
WHIP   *½ pint heavy cream*
2 packets Equal or Sweet'N Low
TOP each serving of pudding with a generous dollop of sweetened cream and dust the top with a dash of unsweetened cocoa or cinnamon.

Serves 4.

Nutritional Values per Serving

Carbohydrate	8.7 gms
Protein	4.4 gms
Calories	282
Fat	25.0 gms
Fiber	0.0 gms

Strawberry Preserves

. . . . this surprisingly simple recipe has a taste light-years beyond the commercially available "dietetic" jellies and jams. Great on Colonial light toast, or as a topping for sugar-free cheesecake or puddings. Once again, thanks to Bill Parker for this one.

RINSE, STEM, and QUARTER   *1 qt fresh strawberries*
PLACE into saucepan.
ADD   *juice of 1 lemon*
COVER and SIMMER until berries soften and give up their juice.

Meanwhile, in a separate bowl:
DISSOLVE   *2 envelopes unflavored gelatin*
for 1 minute in   *½ cup water*
ADD gelatin mixture to berries and REMOVE from heat.

With electric mixer on low speed:
MIX IN   *10 packets Equal or Sweet'N Low*
POUR into storage jar or container.
REFRIGERATE uncovered for 2 hours, then STIR WELL, and
    COVER.
REFRIGERATE AGAIN for at least 12 hours to set.
USE as needed. Store in refrigerator.

MAKES about 64 servings of 1 tablespoon each.

Nutritional Values per Serving

Carbohydrate	0.9 gms
Protein	0.1 gms
Calories	5
Fat	less than 0.1 gms
Fiber	0.2 gms

10

Fat, Fiber, Fortitude . . . and Eskimos?

*N*OW that you have gone through the weight-loss phase and made your transition onto maintenance, you should be reveling in your new, slimmer body. And if you are like most of my patients, you are feeling better and more energetic than you have in years. You should be getting into the swing of the low-carbohydrate lifestyle and discovering just how much you can enjoy foods that you never thought allowable on a diet. You should not only be preparing and enjoying the recipes found in the previous chapter, but be experimenting on your own and delighting in finding ways to convert many of your favorite foods into low-carbohydrate delicacies. But despite all this, you may have some doubts about the long-term consequences of the low-carbohydrate dietary lifestyle to your health.

Unfortunately, your doubts won't be much assuaged by what you read in most newspapers and magazines. As we discussed before, today's dieter—and even nondieter—is much more health conscious than ever before, and this fact is not lost on today's publishers—they know that health information sells. The problem is that much of the information is contradictory, and, in many cases, outright misleading. In this chapter, we will examine the issues that are currently much in vogue in the publishing world, their scientific basis (or lack thereof), and correlate them to the PSMF and our low-carbohydrate maintenance plan. We will deal with the following "hot topics," most of which practically jump out at you just about every time you open the pages of a magazine or newspaper:

- cholesterol
- fiber
- fish oil
- monounsaturated fatty acids
  (one that is soon to be "hot")

You will learn about cholesterol—the main concern on almost everyone's mind these days—and its various components, and about how cholesterol lab tests can sometimes be misleading. And although the discussion of the effects of the low-carbohydrate diet on cholesterol levels will be held off until the next chapter, you will learn now about the effects fiber, fish oil, and monounsaturated fatty acids exert on your blood cholesterol and your general health, and how to use them as a part of your maintenance program. Also, you will discover a way—by asking a single question—to sort through all the latest "medical breakthroughs" and separate the truly valid from the ones that need more investigation before being blindly followed. To get started, let's look at the recent history of fiber, fish oil, and monounsaturated fats.

Since 1972, when a famous paper was published correlating the high levels of fiber in the diet of certain African tribespeople with their low levels of colon cancer and other "diseases of civilization," there has been a mad rush on the part of health-conscious people everywhere to increase their consumption of fiber. Over the past few years, many medical papers as well as many articles in the lay press have described a type of fatty acid—Omega-3 fatty acid—found mainly in certain cold-water fish, the consumption of which is purported to decrease serum cholesterol and perhaps decrease the incidence of heart disease. Sales of Omega-3 fatty acids in the form of fish oil supplements are booming.

Much more recently, several prestigious medical journals have published research articles that indicate that the increased consumption of monounsaturated fats, such as olive oil, not only lowers serum cholesterol but lowers high blood pressure and brings about better control of diabetes. As of this writing, the demand for monounsaturated oils hasn't yet skyrocketed, but based upon past history, it wouldn't be a bad idea to buy stock in the olive-oil processing industry. What does this evidence mean to you the dieter and presumably, the health-conscious individual? Should you consume bowls of bran and handfuls of fish-oil pills while swilling olive oil by the cup? Let's look at fiber and the different types of fats and oils a little more closely, and derive a plan of supplementation—if necessary —to help improve our health while maintaining our weight.

Cholesterol

Since so much of the research on Omega-3 fatty acids (O-3 FA), monounsaturated fatty acids, and fiber relates to their effect on cholesterol, let's examine this business of raising or lowering the levels of cholesterol and see what it really means. What are the HDLs, LDLs, VLDLs, and triglycerides that we read so much about? What actually is cholesterol, and what does it do?

Cholesterol, a lipid, is a waxy substance that is the precursor of all naturally occurring steroids—corticosteroids, sex hormones, bile acids, and vitamin D—synthesized by the body. As discussed in Chapter 3, cholesterol is also a structural lipid in that it is an integral part of cell membranes, nerve linings, and other body components. Of the cholesterol found in the blood, about one-fourth to one-half comes from the average diet, while the remainder is manufactured by the body from synthesis that occurs in the liver (50%), in the intestines (15%), and the remainder (35%) in the skin and other tissues. After its synthesis, cholesterol is released into the blood and is transported to its different destinies by various lipoproteins.

Lipoproteins are molecular structures made of lipids and proteins packaged together that bind with cholesterol and carry it through the blood. While there are several different lipoproteins that scientists have identified, we will be concerned with the three that are most commonly measured. Ranging from the smallest to the largest, they are high density lipoprotein (HDL), low density lipoprotein (LDL), and very low density lipoprotein (VLDL).

- *VLDL* carries triglycerides (fat molecules) in the blood. VLDL also has the ability to be converted rapidly into LDL, the main carrier of cholesterol in the bloodstream.

- *LDL* usually transports the cholesterol from its place of synthesis and delivers it to the areas where it is incorporated into cell membranes or used to synthesize steroid hormones. Unfortunately, LDL also delivers cholesterol to the arterial walls where it can be deposited as plaque and ultimately result in arterial narrowing and heart disease.

- *HDL,* the so-called good cholesterol, removes cholesterol from the tissues and transports it back to the liver, where it is converted into bile acids and discharged into the intestine.

When we have our total cholesterol measured, the number we get back from the lab represents the total amount of cholesterol circulating in our blood including all that which is bound to LDL, VLDL, and HDL. If our total cholesterol is high, that could be bad for us, or not so bad, depending upon the various amounts of the different lipoproteins that the total comprises. If our cholesterol is high because we have much greater than normal amounts of HDL, we are in good shape. If, however, we find our total cholesterol to be low, we need—before we congratulate ourselves on being at decreased risk for heart disease—to make sure that it is not low because we have abnormally low amounts of HDL. The point is that a blood test result that shows only the total cholesterol is not the best indicator of our blood lipid status, because as most physicians now know, a high or low serum cholesterol doesn't tell us much without our knowing what subunits it's made of. If, for example, you came to my office as a patient, and I found your total serum cholesterol to be very elevated, I would strongly suspect that you would have an increased risk for heart disease—but I wouldn't know for certain unless I checked your LDL and HDL as well.

To better assess our degree of risk, we should get a "fraction-ated" cholesterol test, which is one that gives us not only total cholesterol, but all the lipoprotein components or "fractions" as well. With these results in hand, we can much more accurately predict our degree of risk for heart disease, since the less total cho-lesterol that we have relative to our HDL (good cholesterol), the better off we are. We can use that ratio as a measure of our coronary risk level—with anything less than 4 being good, and the lower, the better. If, for example, we have a total cholesterol of 180 (a low figure), but have an HDL of only 30, our total–cholesterol-to-HDL ratio would be 180 divided by 30, or 6—a fairly high ratio. On the other hand, if our total cholesterol was 270 (a number that would get the attention of most physicians), but our HDL was 90, you can see that our ratio would be 270 over 90, or 3, which would indicate that our risk for heart disease would be less than average—even in the face of a high total cholesterol.

Now that we have an idea of what the different cholesterol subunits are and what they do in our blood, we will be better able to understand the way that different diets, medicines, and the fat and fiber food components alter the ratios of these subunits to change the degree of risk for heart disease. Since we know that a lower total–cholesterol-to-HDL ratio is better, let's see how can we bring that about. There are several ways. We can decrease our total cholesterol while keeping our HDL the same, which will decrease the ratio. We can maintain our total cholesterol level where it is while increasing our HDL fraction and produce an identical result. We can undertake some regimen whereby we decrease both our total cholesterol and HDL, but decrease the HDL less, and improve our ratio.

The LDL or "bad cholesterol" fraction when compared to the HDL can also be used to predict the degree of risk for heart disease—the LDL over HDL ratio is optimal at 3 or under. So, we can decrease our risk factors by increasing HDL relative to LDL in the same way as when compared to total cholesterol—by raising HDL levels while keeping LDL the same, or by decreasing LDL while maintaining the same serum level of HDL.

Now that we know that it is the two ratios—total cholesterol to HDL, and LDL to HDL—that are important and not simply increased or decreased levels of total cholesterol, we can examine the ways that fiber, O-3 fatty acids, and monounsaturated fatty acids bring about changes in these ratios and consequently reduce, increase, or have no effect on the risk of heart disease. But before we forge ahead, let's look at some interesting facts about cholesterol—some that you're probably aware of, and some that may surprise you.

As we discuss the following points, you should be aware that when many of the studies were done that provided much of the information we know today about the role of cholesterol in heart disease, only total cholesterol was studied—only recently have researchers been regularly using cholesterol subunits in their investigations. Although we saw above that total cholesterol alone is not the best indicator of blood lipid status, it has been a valuable research tool. The reason for this is that *usually* an elevated serum cholesterol is caused by an elevated level of LDL along with decreased or normal levels of HDL. Thus, increased total cholesterol implies an increased ratio of LDL to HDL, and this case generally holds true.

If a researcher has a study population of subjects, all of whom have markedly elevated levels of serum cholesterol, odds are that most of them will have high total-cholesterol/LDL-to-HDL ratios. If the researcher gives them a drug and their total cholesterol—the only thing measured—falls, and they then subsequently have a decreased rate of heart disease compared to a control group of subjects that didn't receive the drug and didn't lower their total cholesterol, the case can be made that lowering total cholesterol reduces the incidence of heart disease. We know now that the lipoprotein ratio change is what brought about this decreased risk, but in the precise terms of these studies, it is attributed to the lowering of total serum cholesterol. So, throughout this book, whenever I refer to lower serum cholesterol levels causing a particular effect, what I mean is that the reduction in the lipoprotein ratios caused whatever effect we happen to be discussing.

From the multitude of studies done on cholesterol, the following relationships between heart disease, diet, and cholesterol levels have fairly conclusively been shown:

• patients with genetic diseases that cause them to have tremendously elevated levels of cholesterol have a high incidence of early, severe heart disease.

• atherosclerosis (plaque buildup in the arteries) can be produced in animals by increasing the level of cholesterol in their blood.

• high cholesterol levels correlate directly with increased incidence of heart disease in humans.

• lowering elevated cholesterol levels by the use of drugs produces a decreased incidence of heart disease.

The following relationships have been demonstrated in medical studies, but not as conclusively as have the preceding:

• increased intake of saturated fat in the absence of corresponding carbohydrate reduction usually leads to an increase in cholesterol levels—but not in all studies; some show no change.

• increased intake of cholesterol leads to increased levels of serum cholesterol. Again, not in all cases. In fact, in about two-thirds of the cases there is no increase at all.

To summarize what we know from these studies, we can say that high serum cholesterol definitely leads to an increased rate of heart disease, and that by reducing elevated cholesterol levels, we can reduce the rate of heart disease. We can also say that by increasing the amount of saturated fat in our diet, and perhaps by increasing our intake of cholesterol, we can increase our blood cholesterol level. Conversely, if we reduce our intake of saturated fat and perhaps cholesterol, we can reduce our blood cholesterol levels. In simplest terms, if we eat more fat, our blood cholesterol rises; if our blood cholesterol rises, we are at greater risk for heart disease. Therefore, if we eat more fat, we increase our risk of heart disease, correct? Not necessarily. In one of the fascinating inconsistencies of medicine, this has not been shown.

In several large studies comparing the levels of saturated fat intake of certain populations of people—in some cases, entire cities—with the prevalence of heart disease, no correlation was found. In one such study reported in the *British Journal of Medicine* in 1988, the reverse was the case. In one city in England, the population consumed a much greater amount of saturated fat than did the people in another city of the same size and socioeconomic makeup, yet suffered much less heart disease. So, even though A leads to B, and B leads to C, there is no conclusive evidence that A leads to C—at least not in the case of increased consumption of fat leading to heart disease.

I don't want you to get the wrong idea, however. I am not advocating that you start eating lard by the plateful in an effort to decrease your risk of heart disease. I'm just trying to demonstrate the state of medical knowledge on this subject at this point. I do believe that we should do everything we can to decrease our cholesterol levels—more specifically, our total-cholesterol and/or LDL to HDL ratios—and a low-carbohydrate diet will do this by decreasing the synthesis of cholesterol in our bodies. We will examine the way this works in the next chapter, and shortly we will look at how fiber, O-3 fatty acids, and monounsaturated fatty acids affect our cholesterol levels while providing other health benefits as well. But before we finish with cholesterol, let's ask this question: Can cholesterol levels be too low? Everyone is always concerned about abnormal cholesterol elevation, but what about the opposite?

Can Cholesterol Be Too Low?

A recent study in a prestigious medical journal, *The Lancet,* demonstrated that men and, to a lesser degree, women who have very low cholesterol levels appear to be afflicted with a great deal more cancer than their counterparts who have normal or slightly elevated serum cholesterol levels. Patients in similar studies not only developed cancer at a more frequent rate, but they developed cancers that were extremely malignant and deadly. Pondering these findings, some researchers have speculated that the low levels of cholesterol in these patients may have caused their cell membranes to have become weakened, thus allowing easier invasion by the cancer cells. Whatever the reason, scientists will probably find that there is an optimal range of serum cholesterol that will result in neither an increased rate of heart disease nor an increased rate of cancer formation. Based upon the heart-disease/cholesterol studies, the upper range should probably be around 200, and based on *The Lancet* study mentioned above, the lower level should be around 170–180. Interestingly, both the PSMF and the low-carbohydrate maintenance diet keep the serum cholesterol levels of most people in this range.

Fiber

We touched on fiber in Chapter 3, and again in Chapter 8 where we learned how to increase our fiber intake by choosing foods with a low effective carbohydrate content. Now let's look at fiber in a little more detail, putting emphasis on the various alterations the consumption of fiber produces in our bodies. There are two main categories of fiber—soluble and insoluble. Soluble fiber dissolves in water; insoluble fiber does not. Ironically, the effect that most people (including the original researchers) associate with fiber—increased frequency of bulky, soft stools—is the effect caused by the least metabolically active fiber, insoluble fiber. Soluble fiber generates both of the positive metabolic benefits brought about by fiber— lower cholesterol and blood sugar stabilization.

Insoluble fiber, composed of cellulose, lignins, and some hemicelluloses, is found in high concentration in wheat bran products, whereas soluble fiber, composed of pectin, gums, and certain storage starches, is found in oat bran, fruits, vegetables, and psyllium husks (psyllium husks comprise the majority of the fiber in Konsyl, Metamucil, and other commercial bulking laxatives). In many cases, soluble and insoluble fiber will be found together in food items, but usually one kind will predominate. These fibers have different mechanical effects that you can demonstrate easily with a simple experiment.

Go to the grocery store and purchase some unprocessed wheat bran—sometimes called miller's bran—along with a container of Konsyl, or if that's not available, Metamucil. The wheat bran is primarily insoluble fiber, while the Konsyl or Metamucil is made of soluble fiber. At home, stir two tablespoons of the wheat bran into one glass of water and then stir two tablespoons of the Konsyl or Metamucil into another glass of water. Leave them alone for fifteen minutes then come back and observe the difference. Although there will be a little fiber in suspension in the water, the great mass of the wheat bran will have settled to the bottom of its glass pretty much unchanged. The glass containing the Konsyl, however, will be filled with a thick, gelatinous glob of fiber expanded with the water it has absorbed—if you turn the glass over, this glob probably won't even fall out.

This experiment demonstrates basically what happens in your digestive tract. When you eat a large amount of insoluble fiber— wheat bran, for instance—it passes through your intestines and colon fairly quickly and relatively intact, although it does absorb a little water as it goes through, which adds bulk to the stool. Soluble fiber, as you might imagine after viewing the experiment with the glasses of water, acts differently. As it absorbs water, it forms a viscous gel that slows the transit through the digestive system and doesn't pass through unchanged. In the colon, the soluble fiber gel is acted upon by the resident bacteria and partially fermented, producing among other things, gas. The expansion of this gas can cause some abdominal discomfort, more about which later. Aside from the differences in the two fibers in terms of their mechanical passage through the digestive tract, there are great differences in their metabolic effects, with soluble fiber being the metabolically active fiber.

Soluble fiber has two metabolic effects, which it brings about in several different ways. The first is its ability to stabilize the erratic fluctuations of blood sugar caused by the consumption of a meal containing large quantities of simple sugars. This effect—which is helpful to diabetics and is the basis for the "fiber hypothesis" in the treatment of this disease—is due to several properties of the soluble fiber. The gel that is formed enmeshes the gastric contents and slows the absorption of the glucose, preventing rapid rises in blood glucose. Also, this increased viscosity decreases the absorption of carbohydrate from the small intestine, and in a way not entirely known, it affects the functioning of certain digestive enzymes, which results in a further slowing of the absorption of carbohydrates.

These effects can be helpful in the management of diabetes since the slower the sugars are absorbed, the less rapidly blood glucose levels rise, and consequently, the less insulin is required. This blunting effect on blood glucose elevations has given rise to the current method of dietary management for diabetics in which patients are encouraged to consume large quantities of complex carbohydrates. Many people seem to believe that there is something magical about complex carbohydrates that improves the diabetic condition, but in fact, it is the soluble fiber content of the complex carbohydrates that exerts the positive effect on blood glucose. Clever experiments have been done in which the typical complex-carbohydrate diet was broken down into its two components—carbohydrates and fiber. When the combination was given to diabetics, their blood glucose was stabilized. When the fiber component alone was given, the blood glucose was similarly stabilized, but when the carbohydrate component alone was given, the patients' blood glucose levels shot up erratically. This research has shown, I think conclusively, that it is the soluble fiber component of the complex carbohydrates that produces all the beneficial effects of complex-carbohydrate diets. The combination of fiber supplements such as Konsyl or Metamucil and a low-carbohydrate diet, in my opinion, offers the best dietary treatment for diabetes.

How about nondiabetics? Does soluble fiber help them? I think so, because soluble fiber, even in the nondiabetic person, slows the absorption of carbohydrates and therefore produces a much less elevated insulin response. As we have discussed in Chapter 3, and will discuss again in detail in Chapter 11, chronically elevated insulin levels can produce many harmful effects, and anything that we can do to reduce these insulin levels has a positive effect on our health. Soluble fiber is probably helpful in the nondiabetic individual, and certainly not harmful, so there is no reason not to consume it. Later in this section I will explain how you can easily supplement your diet with soluble fiber.

The second metabolic effect visited upon people who consume soluble fiber is a decrease in their lipoprotein ratios, and as a result, a lower risk for heart disease. A recent study demonstrated that when subjects added as little as 10 grams per day (3 teaspoons of Metamucil) of soluble fiber to their diets, they reduced their total serum cholesterol by as much as 17 percent, while not affecting their HDL levels. This, of course, reduced their total cholesterol-to-HDL ratio—a beneficial effect. Further investigation has revealed that soluble fiber does indeed reduce the levels of cholesterol by reducing the levels of LDL.

Soluble fiber induces this cholesterol-lowering in a couple of ways. First, it binds with bile acids in the intestines and prevents their reabsorption. Earlier in this chapter, we discussed how cholesterol is transported by HDL to the liver, where it is converted to bile acids and discharged into the intestine. These bile acids help to emulsify fats to aid in their digestion, and they are then reabsorbed, carried to the liver, and discharged again as needed. When soluble fiber binds these bile acids and prevents their reabsorption, the liver has to convert more cholesterol to bile acids, and thus, blood levels of cholesterol are lowered. Second, there is some evidence that soluble fiber may actually decrease the synthesis of LDL in the intestine, while at the same time increasing the synthesis of HDL. Obviously, this effect would change the LDL to HDL ratio in a positive way.

It should be apparent that increasing our consumption of fiber—especially soluble fiber—is beneficial to us. It stabilizes our blood glucose, decreases serum insulin levels, decreases serum cholesterol, and changes our lipoprotein ratios for the better. Let's see how we can increase our intake of fiber on our low-carbohydrate maintenance plan.

Increasing Fiber Intake

Before we start trying to increase our fiber intake, let's determine some level to shoot for. How much fiber is enough? Several surveys have shown that the average American consumes somewhere in the neighborhood of 10 to 12 grams of fiber per day. Most nutritionists, however, recommend *at least* 25 grams per day, except in certain states such as obstructive bowel disorders. In January 1985, Drs. Eaton and Konner published an interesting article in the *New England Journal of Medicine* that described their research into the composition of the diet of prehistoric man. Their contention (with which I agree) is that the human body developed a digestive system to make the best use of the foods available in those early times. There has been very, very little, if any, change in the human body over the past forty thousand years, but there has been considerable change in the diet fed to it. The authors believe that if we could consume a diet today that more closely approximates the diet of our primitive ancestors, we would be much the healthier for our efforts, since our ancient relatives didn't fall prey to diabetes, heart disease, and other diseases of modern man. They state that Paleolithic man consumed about 50 grams of fiber per day. (These same authors along with Marjorie Shostak have recently published a book entitled *The Paleolithic Prescription* that updates their research. Based on new findings, they have revised their estimate of the fiber content of primitive man's diet upward from 50 grams per day (the figure in their original article) to 100–150 grams per day. Americans now consume 10 grams of fiber per day, the nutritionists advise we should at least consume 25 grams per day, and here is recent evidence that we should perhaps consume much more—even up to 150 grams per day. What should we do? I feel that 50 to 60 grams per day is probably more than adequate, and that level of intake can easily be achieved. If you follow the maintenance diet outlined in Chapter 8 and eat around 50–60 grams per day of nonfiber carbohydrate (50–60 ECC grams), you will consume from 20 to 40 grams of fiber daily. You can augment that with 10 to 20 grams more by taking either Konsyl or Metamucil, which I recommend if you have any sort of cholesterol problems. I also recommend that you add additional fiber in this form to the PSMF if you are having difficulty with bowel irregularity.

Konsyl has the most fiber per dose (6 grams per teaspoon) of any I've found. It contains no carbohydrates and can easily be mixed with a glass of Diet Tang, Crystal Light, or other similar beverage. Metamucil and all the others I have found contain 3.4 grams of fiber per teaspoon and can be mixed in the same way as Konsyl. Be careful that you choose the sugar-free versions of any of these you may purchase since most brands have a sweetened variety. I find it easiest to drink a glass of sugar-free Tang mixed with a couple of teaspoons of Konsyl each morning and evening as a part of my daily routine. This gives me an extra 24 grams of soluble fiber daily to add to the 20 to 40 grams I get in my diet.

A few words of caution. Drink the mixture as soon as you shake it or stir it up. If you let it sit, you will end up with the slimy, gelatinous mess we discussed earlier. Also, don't jump into this fiber supplementation with a lot of gusto. It takes your digestive tract a while to adjust to the increased fiber load. When I read the Paleo-lithic-nutrition article in the *New England Journal of Medicine* in 1985, I became convinced that I needed to increase my intake of fiber. Never one for cautious restraint, I started taking a spoonful of a fiber supplement every time I thought about it. My fiber intake increased to about 100 grams per day within 24 hours, and I soon regretted my haste. I was soon afflicted with severe abdominal cramping, bloating, and outright nausea. What was worse was that it took a couple of days for my symptoms to diminish. So, learn once again from my bad example. Start with your maintenance diet, which will probably provide more fiber than you're used to, and then progress to fiber supplementation very slowly.

Omega-3 Fatty Acids

Nearly everyone by now has heard of many of the health benefits attributed to an increased intake of Omega-3 fatty acids. This fat, usually found in high concentration in certain fish oils, has been said to decrease the rate of heart attack, improve skin conditions, cure arthritis, thin the blood, reduce high blood pressure, and lower serum cholesterol levels. Does it really do these things? Are the claims that this is a wonder drug (or food) valid? Let's look at what the research has shown on O-3 fatty acids and see if they are a valuable addition to the PSMF and to our maintenance plan.

What exactly are O-3 fatty acids? In Chapter 3, we discussed polyunsaturated fatty acids and how they are made of chains of carbon atoms connected by both single and double carbon-carbon bonds. O-3 FA is a fatty acid that is made of 20 carbons with 5 double bonds. By scientific convention, the end carbon of the chain is called the omega carbon, and the first double bond found—count-ing from the omega carbon—in O-3 FA is on the third carbon, or carbon number 3. Thus, O-3 FAs are a family of polyunsaturated fats all with a double bond on the third carbon from the end and four other double bonds elsewhere in the chain. The particular O-3 FA in this family that has been studied the most and that seems to produce the beneficial effects is one with the unwieldy name of *eicosapentaenoic acid (EPA)*. Another important fatty acid that we will study in this chapter is not an Omega-3, but an Omega-6 fatty acid called *gamma linolenic acid (GLA)*. (Omega-6 fatty acids have their first double bond on the sixth carbon from the end.)

It has long been known that Eskimos and certain other groups of people, despite a diet high in fat, have a low incidence of atherosclerosis and heart disease. In the mid-1970s researchers studied this phenomenon and found that although Eskimos did indeed eat a diet high in fat, they also consumed 5 to 10 grams of EPA daily. Furthermore, when these same Eskimos moved into town and adopted a more Western lifestyle including a diet containing little EPA, they began suffering more heart disease—ultimately having heart attacks at about the same rate as their Western counterparts. It appears that this increased amount of EPA in the rural Eskimo diet offers some protective benefit against heart disease.

Many people assume that the large quantities of EPA in the Eskimo diet come from the fish that they eat, but this is not entirely true. EPA is not synthesized by fish at all, but instead by certain plankton found in very cold northern waters. The fish found in these northern regions eat this plankton and concentrate the EPA in their fat. Seals and walruses—the mainstay of the Eskimo diet along with whale meat and blubber—eat these fish in great amount, concentrating the amount of EPA even further. Thus, adding fish to your diet doesn't necessarily add EPA to your diet. To increase your intake of EPA, you must eat fish from very cold waters (herring, chinook salmon, or mackerel) where the plankton that produce EPA are found, or you must increase the amount of seal and walrus meat in your diet. Or more reasonably, you can take EPA supplements. A little later I'll tell you the best way to add these supplements to your diet.

Gamma linolenic acid (GLA), found in certain fairly uncommon plant seeds, is another fatty acid—an Omega-6 fatty acid—that provides many of the same health benefits as does EPA. In fact, GLA actually has more cardioprotective properties than does EPA, and both consumed together are much more potent than either alone. Mother's milk, the perfect food, contains large amounts of both EPA and GLA, which are used by the growing child. Since, once off breast milk, our diets contain little GLA, we have enzymes that can convert other dietary fatty acids into GLA (and EPA also). But as we age, these enzymes become much less active, requiring that we get our GLA and EPA from more direct sources. Also, stress and increased consumption of alcohol, hydrogenated oils, and refined sugars decrease the effectiveness of these converting enzymes, further increasing our need for direct supplementation. Before discussing these supplements, however, let's look at how these fatty acids actually work to protect us from heart disease.

Prostaglandins

Prostaglandins, compounds that are produced from both Omega-6 and Omega-3 fatty acids, act as biochemical messengers that regulate many body systems at the cellular level—notably, the cardiovascular system and the immune system. In fact, most medicines—aspirin and ibuprofen, to name two—that decrease inflammation and reduce pain, work by acting to decrease the body's production of the particular prostaglandins that are responsible for those injurious effects. The prostaglandins that regulate these systems usually are of two kinds—one that increases a certain effect and one that decreases the same effect. Depending upon the effect we are talking about, these prostaglandins could be called "good" prostaglandins or "bad" prostaglandins. Using pain as an example, prostaglandins that increase pain would be "bad" prostaglandins; conversely, those that decrease pain would be "good" prostaglandins.

Prostaglandins, both good and bad, have several effects on the cardiovascular system that we can modify by our intake of the O-3 fatty acid EPA and the O-6 fatty acid GLA. Prostaglandins can increase or inhibit the ability of *platelets* to aggregate, and they can promote or discourage the constriction of arteries (*vasoconstriction*). To better understand how these prostaglandin-produced effects bring about better cardiovascular health, let's look briefly at the genesis of a heart attack.

Heart Attack

Heart attacks (myocardial infarctions) and angina pectoris (severe, crushing chest pain) differ only in the end result—some degree of permanent heart-muscle damage—and are brought about by a narrowing or occlusion of the arteries (coronary arteries) carrying blood to the heart muscle. This narrowing can be caused by a buildup of plaque in the coronary arteries or by spasm of these arteries or by a combination of the two. The most common cause is the plaque buildup combined with some spasm. Where does this plaque come from?

Most physicians agree that the first step in the formation of plaque is some kind of injury to the inner wall of the artery. This is one of the ways in which smoking is thought to contribute to heart disease, because nicotine causes damage to the arterial lining. Once the damage occurs, the body sets in motion a repair process that basically consists of a scab formation at the site of the injury. Certain clotting components present in the blood make a kind of mesh around the injury, and other blood components called platelets aggregate at the site and form the clot. As the clot grows, it catches cholesterol circulating in the blood and incorporates it into the grow- ing mass—referred to as plaque—on the arterial wall. With time, this process continues, and the plaque grows until it reaches a size large enough to reduce dramatically the amount of blood that can flow through the artery. The plaque can also irritate the artery and make it more prone to spasm and constrict, shutting down the blood supply even more.

When this arterial narrowing caused by plaque, or by a com- bination of plaque and constriction, decreases the supply of oxygen- rich blood to the heart below a critical level, severe heart pain occurs. This heart pain, crushing in intensity, is accompanied by profuse sweating, inability to get enough air, and usually a cold, mottled- gray skin color. If the oxygen is restored to the heart muscle be- fore any damage takes place, the pain usually diminishes and the patient is said to have had an attack of angina. If, however, the heart muscle is deprived of oxygen for a long enough period of time, the muscle is permanently damaged, and the patient has suffered a heart attack.

Unfortunately for many people, their first heart attack is also their last, because they don't survive it. The heart beats in a syn- chronous fashion due to an electric impulse that spreads through the heart tissue, causing the heart-muscle cells to contract in a co- ordinated fashion that results in blood's being pumped throughout the body. If the narrowing caused by plaque happens to be in an artery that feeds an area of the heart critical to the transmission of this regulatory electrical impulse, the rhythmic beating of the heart can cease. When the heart ceases to beat for even a few minutes, or beats erratically in a manner that doesn't pump blood, the patient dies.

Where do EPA, GLA, and prostaglandins fit into this picture? Both EPA and GLA are precursors in the formation of prostaglandins that (1) inhibit the aggregation of platelets, and (2) tend to decrease the degree of vasoconstriction. Another fatty acid in the blood, ar- achidonic acid, is a precursor for prostaglandins that do the exact opposite and promote both platelet aggregation and vasoconstriction. The GLA is converted through an intermediate form—D-homo gamma linolenic acid (DGLA)—to a prostaglandin that inhibits platelet aggregation and vasoconstriction. But ironically, DGLA can also be further converted by the body into arachidonic acid—the precursor to the bad prostaglandins. While the EPA partially inhibits the transformation of arachidonic acid into the harmful prostaglandins, it plays its major role in preventing the formation of arachidonic acid from DGLA. It is this balance of DGLA to arachidonic acid that determines cardiovascular health. Thus, increased consumption of EPA and GLA shifts the prostaglandin control system in a direction that keeps the heart arteries open and prevents platelets from aggregating and helping to form the plaque.

In addition to beneficially manipulating the prostaglandin control system, O-3 FAs reduce the incidence of heart disease by other means as well. O-3 FAs reduce the level of triglycerides in the blood, they often reduce the serum cholesterol, they increase the oxygen supply to the tissues, and they thin the blood. Because of this host of positive effects, I think that the proper use of O-3 FA and GLA supplements is indicated for most people as a preventative measure against heart disease. In addition, as far as the PSMF is concerned, some recent research has shown that during diets such as the PSMF, the body's supplies of O-3 FAs (but not other fatty acids) are depleted and should be replenished via supplementation. Before you launch off to the pharmacy and load yourself with fish oil capsules, there are several questions that must be answered. What kind of supplements should I get—will any fish oil capsules fill the bill? How much should I take? Are there any side effects?

Fatty Acid Supplementation

As you have probably expected, nothing that seems this good can be without problems. The main problems concerning fatty acid supplementation are (1) the quality of the supplements readily available, and (2) due to the dosage required to obtain the desired benefits, the possibility of oversupplementing. Let's look at these problems in more detail.

The O-3 FAs, due to their high degree of unsaturation, are prone to oxidation and rancidity. This means that they don't have a particularly long shelf life (although once in the gelatin capsules, they remain stable if stored between 60 and 78 degrees). The most important factor in their stability, however, is the quality of oil that goes into the capsule to begin with. I have seen laboratory analyses of various fish oil supplements that have considerably less active O-3 FA than described on the label due to this oxidation process—or to poor quality control prior to encapsulation. Certain ingredients such as vitamin E can be added to the supplements to help slow this process, but often the wrong form of vitamin E is used. Also, fish concentrate PCB, heavy metals, and other pollutants in their fat. When manufacturers process cold-water fish to extract fish oil for use in supplements, often they are unable to remove all these pollutants. For this reason alone, you must use caution in your selection of a fatty acid supplement. Finally, fish oil supplements alone provide only EPA and no GLA, which is thought by many to be a more potent cardioprotective agent than EPA.

Since fatty acids are not really a drug but a food supplement, they need to be taken in large doses to fully deliver their benefits. Most literature on the subject recommends that patients take 10 to 20 capsules daily to accomplish the desired benefits. With these dosages some problems can develop. One of the beneficial effects of O-3 FA is the thinning of the blood, and this can be overdone to the point that bleeding becomes a problem. (Let me hurry to point out that the degree of blood thinning brought about by the recommended amount of O-3 FA is approximately equivalent to that of one regular-strength aspirin tablet.) However, Eskimos who ingest huge amounts of O-3 fatty acids have many bleeding problems, and they have a much greater than normal incidence of a type of stroke (hemorrhagic stroke) caused by bleeding into the brain. Medical evidence as to the cause of stroke in Eskimo populations has not clearly implicated only increased dietary EPA—there may be genetic factors as well. In addition, due to the rapidly oxidizing nature of O-3 FAs, there has been some speculation that an increased intake could deplete the body of its supplies of vitamins A, C, and E as well as other antioxidant nutrients and cause a weakening of the immune system. Also some research has shown that diabetic control is much more difficult to achieve in patients taking O-3 fatty acids. Because of these problems, the most prudent course of action, when taking large doses of O-3 only, is to do so under the supervision of your physician.

Which are the best supplements to take? Based on my research in this area, I feel that the supplier of the purest, most active supplements is a company called BioSyn. Their supplements can only be purchased directly from the company. I recommend their OmegaSyn starter pack, which includes both EPA and GLA fatty acids combined into a single supplement capsule, plus another bottle of vitamin and mineral supplements called EFA Enhance that "enhances" the beneficial action of the fatty acids. BioSyn's OmegaSyn supplement is the only one I know that provides both EPA *and* GLA, and that does so in the optimal ratio. By combining EPA and GLA, the dosage of both may be decreased, thereby reducing the risk inherent in taking large doses of EPA alone. You may write or call:

BioSyn
21 Tioga Way
Marblehead, MA 01945
(617) 639-2401
(800) 346-2703

Monounsaturated Fatty Acids

For many years, the prevailing wisdom has been that we should eat diets containing little protein and even less fat. We have been exhorted to consume large amounts of complex carbohydrates and to replace most of the saturated fat in our diet with polyunsaturated fat. If we make these recommended dietary changes (ignoring the fact that the resultant diet is unpalatable to most people for the long term), what kind of health benefits are we likely to see?

There is little doubt that the above-described diet will produce some advantageous changes in our health. It will usually bring about a decrease in blood sugar (if elevated), a decrease in serum insulin levels, a decrease in serum cholesterol, a decrease in LDL, and a slight decrease in HDL (although not as much of a decrease as in the LDL, so the ratio is still improved). Unfortunately, this diet also produces higher levels of serum triglycerides, and if the diet is protein deficient—a risk on a very-low-fat diet—protein malnutrition. There currently exists considerable controversy over the matter of elevated triglycerides. Many physicians consider mildly elevated serum triglycerides to be of no great concern (not so with extremely elevated triglycerides), but everyone generally agrees that the lower the serum triglycerides the better.

A rapidly growing body of recently published research is taking issue with the very-low-fat (mainly polyunsaturated)/high-complex-carbohydrate approach to dieting on several grounds. Numerous researchers are concerned about the high levels of poly-unsaturated fat in many diets because of several animal studies demonstrating that polyunsaturated fatty acids suppress the immune system and increase the risk of developing cancer—probably, again, through increasing the conversion to arachidonic acid, which is immunosuppressive. If you replace saturated fat in your diet with either polyunsaturated fats *or* with monounsaturated fats, you get the same cholesterol/LDL-lowering effects. With monounsaturated fats, however, you don't lower your HDL (in fact, some papers actually show monounsaturated fatty acids to increase HDL levels), and thus you improve your LDL/HDL ratio even more. And mono-unsaturated fats haven't been shown to suppress the immune system or increase cancer formation in laboratory animals in the same way that polyunsaturated fatty acids have. Also, unlike complex carbo-hydrates, monounsaturated fatty acids bring about a significant low-ering of serum triglycerides, thus producing an even better blood lipid profile.

Since monounsaturated fatty acids have more beneficial effects on blood lipid profiles than polyunsaturated fatty acids, and at the same time, no negative effects on the immune system, it makes sense to replace polyunsaturated fats in your diet with mono-unsaturated fats. One major food manufacturer, Procter and Gamble, has already made this move—they have changed their Puritan Oil from a polyunsaturated fat to a monounsaturated fat. You can make this move as well by changing from a vegetable or safflower oil to Puritan Oil or olive oil in your cooking. You may have noticed in the recipe section of the last chapter that virtually all recipes that used oil called for olive oil or canola oil (canola oil or rapeseed oil is the monounsaturated fat in Puritan Oil), and by using these oils you will increase the amount of beneficial monounsaturated fat in your diet. By making your own mayonnaise, you can replace con-siderable saturated fat in your diet with the more healthful mono-unsaturated variety. Commercially prepared mayonnaise, although it contains no carbohydrate, is made from hydrogenated and par-tially hydrogenated oils and as a result contains large amounts of saturated fat. When you prepare it yourself from the recipe in Chap-ter 9, using olive oil or canola oil, you get a monounsaturated mayonnaise that will actually improve your health. (Also, see Ap-pendix B for information about commercially produced canola oil mayonnaise.) You may have to fool with the recipe a little in terms of proportions of the different oils to get the taste and texture that you like, but it is well worth the effort. Using these mono-unsaturated oils is a little more difficult—that's why the commercial people use hydrogenated oil instead. They sacrifice quality for ease of production.

When researchers have used monounsaturated fats in place of complex carbohydrates in the diets of non-insulin dependent diabetics, they have been able to achieve much better control of the patient's blood sugars and insulin levels. We can assume that in normal, nondiabetic subjects, these same benefits would hold true. We have seen earlier in this chapter that the blood sugar/insulin-moderating influence brought about by the consumption of complex carbohydrates comes from the fiber component in the complex—the carbohydrate component alone caused wildly fluctuating blood sugars and elevated insulin levels. Monounsaturated fats (any fats for that matter) cause little, if any, blood sugar and insulin rise, so it is easy to see why substituting monounsaturated fat for carbohydrate would be helpful in the control of diabetes. In the maintenance diet, you are not only replacing carbohydrate with monounsaturated fat, but adding fiber as well. This should be the optimal combination to maintain a healthy blood lipid profile *and* keep your blood sugar and insulin levels in line.

As a means of review, let's lay out in tabular form the effects of the various substances we've studied in this chapter. The effects shown are caused by addition of the particular food component to the diets of research subjects. You must remember that different effects can occur when these substances are consumed in different combinations, and in place of one another in certain diets, e.g., fat/protein for carbohydrate in our maintenance diet.

	cholesterol	LDL	HDL	insulin	blood sugar
saturated fat	↑	↑	↓ =	−	−
EPA & GLA	↓	↓	↑ =	−	−
fiber (soluble)	↓	↓	−	↓	↓
carbohydrates	↓	↓	↓	↑	↑
monounsaturated fat	↓	↓	↑	−	−
polyunsaturated fat	↓	↓	↓ =	−	−

Medical Breakthroughs: How Valid?

There is a single question that you should always ask when you hear or read of the latest medical breakthrough. The question needs to be phrased a little differently depending upon the "breakthrough" involved, so let me use an example to show you what I mean.

Let's invent a hypothetical tribe of Indians called the Wanatabe, who live far from the influences of modern civilization. An intrepid medical researcher spends some time with the Wanatabe and notices that they never seem to be afflicted with cancer of any kind. Our researcher visits a neighboring tribe, the Eedo-Eedos (also hypothetical), and finds them to have the normal amount of cancer that one might expect. He knows that both tribes live in the same climate and follow most of the same customs, yet there is this huge difference in the rate of cancer between them. The first thought our man has is that this disparity can be explained by some hereditary difference in cancer susceptibility between the Wanatabes and the Eedo-Eedos. Upon checking, he finds that it is a fairly common practice for the Wanatabes to marry the Eedo-Eedos and vice versa. He then chases down all the instances of this intermarriage that he can find, and he discovers a startling fact—all the Eedo-Eedos who have come to live with the Wanatabes as new spouses have never gotten cancer, while, conversely, the Wanatabes who have moved in with the Eedo-Eedos have incurred cancer at the same rate as the unfortunate Eedo-Eedos. This fact has not escaped the notice of the Wanatabes, who, in fact, refer to cancer as "Eedo-Nupwithit," which loosely translates to "bad sickness of the Eedo-Eedo."

At this point, our man, who has wisely decided to pitch his tent with the Wanatabe, determines to study the diet of both tribes. He finds, to his amazement, that the diet of both tribes is exactly the same with one exception: the Wanatabes eat a type of bean—the Wanbean—that the Eedo-Eedos never touch. Upon further investigation, he finds that one large family of Eedo-Eedos, however, loves the Wanbean and has traded with the Wanatabe for it regularly throughout many generations. As you have probably guessed, not one person in this Eedo-Eedo family has ever suffered a case of "Eedo-Nupwithit." As he continues his investigation, our researcher confirms that the Wanbean actually does protect against cancer. He gathers his data and heads for civilization with visions of the Nobel prize spinning in his head.

He arrives home and publishes his findings in a prestigious medical journal to the acclaim of his peers. Soon the regular press has picked up on this fantastic discovery and headlines proclaim: "Wanbeans Prevent Cancer!" Companies form to produce the Wanbean in supplement form, and a cancer-fearful public rushes in droves to buy them. You are probably thinking that if the proof were this strong that the Wanbean prevents cancer, you would be rushing to buy the supplements along with everyone else, regardless of price. That may be exactly the correct move to make—but only after you get the answer to the one question that launched us off on this story.

The question is: What *do* the Wanatabe die from? Surely they die. If not, the world would long ago have been overpopulated with Wanatabe. Since this isn't the case, the Wanatabe must die. We need to know what does them in.

If our researcher had done his job properly, he would have found that the Wanatabe live on the average to about the same age as the Eedo-Eedo—close to sixty years old. He would have discovered that most of the Wanatabe died with heart attacks, whereas the Eedo-Eedo never had heart attacks—cancer always got them. He could do all the same studies as before, looking at marriage, etc., and conclude that the Wanbean causes heart disease. The most valuable study he could do would be to try to find a dosage of Wanbean extract that would prevent cancer but not be large enough to cause heart disease. Then we would have cause to celebrate.

The point is that you mustn't accept at face value any statements that you might read or hear without asking what the opposing effects are. If you read that some group of people never get a type of cancer because they eat strawberries, ask what they do get. Make sure that whatever is purported to cure or prevent some particular ailment is not causing something else. In our example above, if not only the Wanatabe but also the Eedo-Eedos who ate the Wanbean had lived on average fifteen years longer than the Eedo-Eedos who did not, then the case could be made for consumption of the Wanbean by everyone.

Let's briefly look at an actual example, although not as extreme, of the Wanbean situation. Earlier in this chapter, I pointed out that Eskimos had a low incidence of heart disease, and good blood lipid profiles in spite of eating diets incredibly high in fat. I explained that this came about because Eskimos ate mainly fish, seal, walrus, and whale meat and blubber, all of which contain large amounts of Omega-3 fatty acids. As in the case of the Wanbean, you could reason that the consumption of O-3 FA supplements in large amounts would decrease your chances of having a heart attack and decide to take these supplements by the handfuls. Before you do, however, ask yourself, "Do Eskimos live forever?" They don't. In fact, Eskimos, compared to non-Eskimos, have a much higher rate of death from both stroke and infections (the latter is probably caused by the decrease in the immune response)—conditions brought about by our friends, the O-3 fatty acids that are in very high concentration in the Eskimo diet.

I'm not trying to dissuade you from taking O-3 FA supplements; I'm telling you to use moderation, and to look at the flip side of any new medical breakthrough. Taking O-3 fatty acids—especially when combined with GLA—in the proper doses provides protection against heart disease and the other problems we previously discussed. Just take them in the doses recommended, and don't overdo it. Don't buy into the fallacy that if a little is good, a lot is better. That's not always the case—especially with medicine.

While I'm on this subject, let me discuss this business of taking aspirin to prevent heart disease. A huge study was recently completed that showed that in males, the taking of *one* regular aspirin every other day dramatically reduced the rate of heart attack. *One regular aspirin every other day.* I can't tell you how many patients I have had that tell me that they take an aspirin every morning and every night. That is too much! Aspirin interferes with the prostaglandin synthesis process, but in *very* low doses. There is even some evidence that too much aspirin negates the positive effects. So, take an aspirin every other day if your physician tells you to—and no more!

We have now seen the benefits of increased consumption of fiber, the O-3 and O-6 fatty acids EPA and GLA, and monounsaturated fats. Some of these substances work by moderating the effects of blood sugar and insulin. In the next chapter we will look in detail at how elevated insulin levels affect many systems of the body, and how the PSMF and the maintenance diet work to moderate the activity of this important hormone in a way that is beneficial to our health.

11

Health Benefits of the PSMF and Maintenance Diet

THE PSMF and the maintenance diet described in this book, if followed, will almost certainly improve your health. You may suspect that the improvement you achieve is the result of the decrease in your weight and percent body fat, and that is partially true—but it is not the entire reason. Along with the positive changes brought about merely by the decrease in amount of body fat, there are three specific benefits you may gain by being on both the PSMF and the maintenance diet:

- reduction in high blood pressure
- reduction in serum cholesterol
- stabilization of erratic blood sugar

As this chapter progresses, you will see how these changes are effected by the regulation and stabilization of your serum insulin levels by low-carbohydrate diets. Also, by learning the scientific basis of these diets, you will gain a better understanding of how most of the minor side effects discussed in the next chapter are caused.

Most physicians generally recognize that obesity—even in the absence of other problems—is a health risk, and that by helping patients reduce their weight, they help them reduce their risk for many diseases. But it is not only the obese who are at risk, and being slender is no guarantee of perfect health.

Think about the people you know who are thin, yet have had heart attacks or high blood pressure or stroke or high cholesterol—or a combination of any of these conditions. Granted, these problems are more common in the overweight, but the overweight don't have the franchise on them. Why is it that when someone who is obese—and is afflicted with this host of maladies—loses weight, he or she generally gets rid of most, if not all, of these risk factors, and yet others, who have never had a weight problem, remain plagued by these problems in spite of their low weight? It appears that there is some risk factor that is increased by gaining weight, decreased by losing weight, and present in many people regardless of whether or not they are overweight.

If we take two groups of people—one group obese, the other nonobese but with high blood pressure and elevated cholesterol—and examine their blood, what do you think we will find? In the obese group, we are certain to find elevated cholesterol, elevated LDL, decreased HDL, increased triglycerides, elevated blood glucose, and elevated serum insulin levels. What about the other group of normal-weight hypertensive subjects—what abnormalities do we find in their blood? *Exactly the same ones that we find in the blood of the obese subjects!* So, nonobese subjects who have the same medical afflictions as the obese—high blood pressure and high cholesterol, for example—often have the same blood profile as the obese. You may think to yourself that if you're going to have these problems anyway, you would rather have them and at least not have the weight problem, too. This is the wrong way to think about it, however, because if you have these problems because you are over-weight, you can get rid of them by losing weight. What do normal-weight people with these afflictions do to get rid of them? Usually, they take medicines prescribed by their doctors to decrease blood pressure and to decrease cholesterol. This attacks the symptoms, but what about the underlying problem? What abnormality do these normal-weight people have that causes them to have the problems generally suffered by the obese?

When overweight people lose their excess fat, they generally end up with lower cholesterol, lower LDL, higher HDL, lower tri-glycerides, lower blood pressure, lower blood sugar, and lower serum insulin levels. If we look at studies that examine these factors individually in normal-weight, hypertensive, hyperlipidemic (having high blood lipids) individuals, what do we find?

We find that we can reduce cholesterol with the use of drugs, but the other problems remain. We can reduce blood pressure, also by using drugs, and sometimes, depending upon the medicine used, cholesterol drops a little, but more often it remains elevated. Blood sugar and insulin levels are so interrelated that it is difficult to affect one without affecting the other; however, in a research setting it can be done. Decreasing blood sugar while keeping insulin levels high seems to have no relationship to any of the other risk factors. But when researchers reduced the serum insulin levels, they found that blood pressure decreased, cholesterol decreased, and the different blood lipid ratios changed for the better. More and more research is being done in this area, and a growing body of evidence now seems to point to elevated levels of serum insulin—a hormone that is vital to life—as the culprit causing the problems found in both the obese and in normal-weight individuals with "obese" blood profiles. Why are these insulin levels elevated? What happens as people gain weight that causes their serum insulin levels to rise? What happens to our insulin levels on the PSMF and on our maintenance diet? To answer these questions, let's look more closely at how insulin works.

The Insulin Connection

As we discussed in Chapter 3, insulin is synthesized in certain cells of the pancreas and released into the blood when blood sugar levels rise. When we consume carbohydrates—especially refined carbohydrates—our blood sugar rises, and insulin is released to transport this sugar from our blood into our cells, where it is stored as glycogen. Insulin transports glucose primarily into the liver cells, but into both muscle and fat cells as well. Researchers don't know the precise means by which insulin achieves this transport, but they speculate that it involves insulin receptors on the walls of the cells. As people gain weight, their fat cells increase in size. This fatty engorgement of the cells stretches the cell wall and deforms the insulin receptors. As these receptors are deformed, they do not work as efficiently, and consequently less blood sugar is transported into the cells. Since less sugar goes into the cells, more remains in the blood, and the blood glucose is higher. Higher blood glucose, through a feedback mechanism, results in the release of more insulin from the pancreas, and the insulin levels continue to climb.

Insulin Resistance

In Chapter 3, we noted that insulin does more than just transport glucose into the cells—insulin also increases the storage of fat. Thus, high insulin levels act to enlarge the fat cells even further, bringing about more stretching of the cell walls, and more distortion of the insulin receptors. This cycle continues, and as the cells become progressively more resistant to insulin, the blood glucose levels increase, stimulating the release of yet more insulin, causing further engorgement of the fat cells, making them even more insulin resistant. If this cycle proceeds, type II diabetes ensues. (This is the paradoxical situation in which the patient has both too much blood sugar *and* too much insulin.) This insulin resistance can occur in normal-weight individuals as well as in the overweight. Many physicians believe that in the normal-weight individual who has this condition there exists some metabolic derangement that brings about insulin resistance (and its resultant problems) as a response to carbohydrate ingestion.

Elevated insulin levels resulting from insulin resistance create a multitude of health problems. Excess insulin causes the kidneys to retain excess sodium, one of the body's electrolytes. Unfortunately, when the kidneys retain sodium, they also retain excess fluid along with it. This means that elevated insulin levels cause fluid retention. (You can see this phenomenon at work in your own body. After you have been on the PSMF and the maintenance diet, your insulin levels will be low. When you arise the morning after your first carbohydrate binge, you will notice that your eyes are swollen, your face is puffy, and you will have difficulty putting on your rings. All due to the fluid retention brought about by the insulin response to your carbohydrate binge.) Excess fluid retention produced by insulin resistance is one of the causes of high blood pressure.

The Insulin-Cholesterol Connection

Cholesterol is synthesized in the body from a substance called acetyl-coenzyme A (Acetyl CoA). Acetyl CoA is produced by many other of the body's biochemical processes and is the start of the cholesterol synthesis chain. As with all substances the body makes, cholesterol synthesis proceeds in a stepwise fashion with the continual building upon and modification of the original substance until the final product—in this case, cholesterol—is produced. Each step along the way is executed by a particular enzyme. (Enzymes are proteins made by the body to do specific jobs. Each enzyme is unique and does only the task for which it is made. Virtually all body repair and synthesis is carried out by enzymes.) In every synthesis chain in the body there is usually one enzyme that controls the rate of synthesis of the particular product, and this is referred to as the rate-limiting enzyme of the sequence in question. In the synthesis of cholesterol, the rate-limiting enzyme is 3-hydroxy-3-methylglutaryl-coenzyme A reductase (HMG CoA Reductase).

The more active HMG CoA Reductase is, the more cholesterol the body makes. And conversely, the less active this enzyme is, the less cholesterol is synthesized. In fact, one of the newer, potent cholesterol-lowering drugs works by inhibiting the activity of this rate-limiting enzyme. Insulin has the opposite effect. It makes HMG CoA Reductase more active, and therefore, elevated insulin levels cause more cholesterol to be produced. Type II diabetics and others with chronically elevated insulin levels typically have high levels of serum cholesterol. By controlling their blood sugar and insulin levels, they can usually gain better control of their high cholesterol levels as well.

In view of the harmful effects described above that are caused by elevated insulin levels and insulin resistance, it is easy to see that any dietary modification we can make that will reduce insulin levels is beneficial. What effect do the PSMF and the maintenance diet have on insulin levels? If we can reduce insulin levels as we diet and maintain, we should gain much more than just a slimmer body.

Insulin Regulation With the PSMF and Maintenance Diet

Aside from the loss of weight, there are three main health benefits produced by the insulin regulation of the PSMF and the low-carbohydrate maintenance diet—lower blood pressure, stabilization of sugar metabolism, and reduced serum cholesterol. These effects are seen on many weight-loss regimens after the weight is lost. On the PSMF, many patients observe these effects very soon —in many cases, long before a significant amount of weight is lost. The reason for this rapid change is that along with losing weight, patients are also quickly lowering their serum insulin levels. Let's look at how the PSMF and maintenance diets lower insulin levels and exactly what that means to us.

As we have discussed, the primary stimulant for the release of insulin into the blood is an increase in the blood sugar level. Blood sugar levels are increased when we eat carbohydrates, especially very refined carbohydrates. And studies have shown that the blood sugar response to the fat/sugar combination and to the protein/sugar combination is much greater than to any of these substances alone. If we eat a typical American diet (loaded with fat, protein, carbohydrate, and calories) first our blood sugar levels and then our insulin levels skyrocket. Remaining on this typical American diet keeps our blood sugar and insulin levels chronically elevated, and if we become insulin-resistant, we develop all the problems we have been discussing.

If, on the other hand, we can reduce our blood sugar, our insulin levels will fall; but how do we reduce our blood sugar levels? We can reduce them effectively with the PSMF and the low-carbohydrate maintenance diet. These diets contain little carbohydrate and therefore allow us to maintain a constant level of blood sugar, which does not stimulate the release of excess insulin. Also, the maintenance diet contains a generous amount of soluble fiber, which even further blunts the blood sugar and insulin response. Without a doubt, these are the most effective diets that I know of to lower blood sugar, decrease insulin levels, and overcome insulin resistance. If you can keep your insulin at normal levels, you should be able to see a marked improvement in your blood pressure and in your serum cholesterol levels.

High Blood Pressure

The PSMF and the maintenance diet are effective in lowering high blood pressure. If you now have high blood pressure and are on medications, you MUST consult with your physician before making any changes in medications or dosages. Many patients who have high blood pressure are taking medicines that are diuretics. These medicines cause them to urinate frequently and thus rid their bodies of the excess fluid in part responsible for their elevated pressure. When patients start the PSMF, due to their reduced carbohydrate intake, in just a few days their insulin levels fall. They notice an almost immediate diuresis as their bodies excrete the excess fluid they have been carrying because of their elevated insulin.

The diuresis you will experience is not entirely due to decreased insulin levels. The ketones formed because of your reduced carbohydrate intake also contribute to the diuresis. Because of this extreme diuresis, people on the PSMF sometimes can become sodium-depleted and even dehydrated. For this reason, it is imperative that you drink at least the required amount of water daily (64 ounces). Also, as you will find in the chapter on side effects, this is probably the only diet you have ever seen that may require you to slightly increase your intake of salt. This addition is sometimes necessary because of the sodium depletion that occurs from the increased diuresis brought about by the fall in insulin levels.

And the process works both ways. Fluid retention (the opposite of diuresis) is responsible for most of the weight gain you will notice after one of your planned "dietary vacations"—especially if the vacation involves the consumption of large amounts of carbohydrates. After being on a low-carbohydrate diet for a period of time, you will become more susceptible to the effects of carbohydrate consumption than you were before starting the diet. If you consume, for example, cake, ice cream, candy, and a nondiet drink at your kid's birthday party, your blood sugar will scream upward, followed in short order by your insulin levels. The elevated insulin levels will cause you to retain fluid, with the resultant aforementioned puffy face, baggy eyes, etc. And this is not to mention the two to four pound water-weight gain you will experience. When you start on your "recovery diet," your insulin levels will drop back to normal, you will urinate away this excess fluid, and you will quickly be back to your old skinny self. But you will have gained firsthand knowledge of what a potent force insulin is.

Although you may view this diuresis as an inconvenience, especially in the early days of the PSMF, you must realize that it is beneficial, and that you are getting rid of excess fluid that your body doesn't actually need. If you happen to have high blood pressure, this diuresis should result in your blood pressure falling to a more normal range.

NOTE: High blood pressure can be caused by several factors in the body other than merely fluid retention. If you have high blood pressure, you must be evaluated by a physician to determine the underlying cause. Only when you know the reason for your high blood pressure will you know the best way to treat it.

Sugar Metabolism Problems

Hypoglycemia, hyperglycemia, prediabetes, borderline diabetes, glucose intolerance—all are names for an inability to properly metabolize dietary sugar. If you have any of these conditions, the PSMF is for you (and so is the maintenance diet). All these conditions are caused by a faulty insulin response to carbohydrate in the diet, and all can be made better by stabilizing the level of blood sugar in the afflicted person. Nothing stabilizes blood sugar better than the PSMF and the low-carbohydrate maintenance diet with its large amount of soluble fiber. IF YOU HAVE TYPE I DIABETES THAT REQUIRES YOU TO TAKE INSULIN, OR TYPE II DIABETES REQUIRING ORAL MEDICATIONS FOR CONTROL, DO NOT UNDERTAKE THIS OR ANY OTHER DIET WITHOUT FIRST CONSULTING YOUR PHYSICIAN.

By consuming a diet that is low in carbohydrate, you allow your body to regulate its blood sugar level via a complex set of internal controls. As blood glucose is needed, your body produces it from its stores of glycogen in a controlled fashion that prevents the erratic gyrations in the blood glucose level that are the hallmarks of many of the above-mentioned disorders. When you dump large amounts of carbohydrate—especially refined carbohydrate—into your system by eating foods that are very sweet, you lose this controlled release of blood glucose, and consequently, your blood glucose levels rise rapidly, engendering a rapid rise in the levels of serum insulin. Depending upon the disorder of carbohydrate metabolism you may have (if any), these insulin levels either go too high too quickly and drive too much blood glucose into the cells, resulting in levels of blood glucose that are too low (hypoglycemia), or the insulin—due to insulin resistance—doesn't do its job, and the blood glucose remains too high (hyperglycemia).

If you adhere first to the PSMF regimen, and then to the maintenance diet, you should never experience the "sugar rushes," dizziness, weakness, faintness, or other symptoms common to people with these disorders of carbohydrate metabolism. As you continue on the maintenance diet, you will feel alert and energetic because you won't have wildly fluctuating blood glucose and insulin levels (nor the problems they cause), though a word of caution is needed.

The longer you stay on a low-carbohydrate maintenance diet, the more sensitive your insulin/blood-glucose control system becomes. Since you will be consuming little actual "active" carbohydrate, and what you do consume will be somewhat blunted by the amount of soluble fiber you eat along with it, your cells will—out of necessity—become very sensitive to insulin; it won't take much to do the job. Whereas before you may have been insulin-resistant, after a time on the maintenance diet, you will be insulin-sensitive. If you eat a large amount of concentrated, refined carbohydrate—an amount you could easily have eaten previously without any symptoms whatsoever—you will probably notice some unpleasant side effects. You may become a little nauseated, dizzy, and/or dysphoric (the medical word for just feeling lousy). These symptoms are brought on by your increased sensitivity to insulin. As you suffer these ill effects, you will decrease the amount of carbohydrate-filled junk food you eat on your—I hope—infrequent binges. My own experience bears this out.

As far as candy is concerned, I can take it or leave it, but not so with pastry. I love all kinds of pastries and other sweet baked goods, and the gooeyer the better. Coffee cakes and sweet rolls with jelly-fruit filling are my favorites. Nothing light and fluffy for me, thank you; I'll take mine sodden with grease and dripping with sugar. At least in the old days I did. On my first binge—after a long while on first the PSMF, then the maintenance diet—I ate ten heavy, glazed, sour-cream, cake doughnuts at one sitting (I told you I wasn't a paragon of restraint). I suffered greatly for this carbohydrate debauch, but the memory of my misery had faded by the time the next dietary vacation came around—I did the same thing, with the same results. It didn't take more than about fifteen or twenty similar episodes until I figured out that the enjoyment I got from stuffing myself with pastries was not worth the price I had to pay afterward. I started to use some restraint, and my eating pattern—even during binges—has changed. You probably think that I'm going to end this story by telling you that I now no longer eat pastries, but such is not the case.

I still eat pastries on my dietary vacations, but believe it or not, I tend more toward the lighter ones now. Also, I eat many more sweet fruits and starchy vegetables that I can't have on my ongoing maintenance diet. I have almost completely eliminated the heavy, rich pastries that I used to love so much. In fact, just writing about them makes me feel a slight twinge of nausea. If every time you try to pet a dog, he bites you, it doesn't take long until you don't care much for the dog. I think that's what has happened to me with very rich desserts and pastries—I guess I've been bitten too often.

My experience is far from unique, as many of my patients have reported similar episodes to me. They think that it is wonderful because they lose their taste for these rich, heavy foods, and then they don't miss what they don't like. By eliminating these items from their diet because of the reactions brought on by increased carbohydrate sensitivity, they have—as a fortunate coincidence— eliminated a huge amount of saturated fat as well.

Elevated Serum Cholesterol

The PSMF and the maintenance diet are typically successful in improving the condition of people who have problems with their levels of blood lipids—this group includes most people who are overweight. One of the ways in which these low-carbohydrate diets effect this positive change, as we discussed earlier in this chapter, is by keeping the insulin levels low and thus decreasing the activity of HMG CoA Reductase (the rate-limiting enzyme in the cholesterol synthesis process). So, by decreasing the activity of this enzyme, our bodies don't synthesize as much cholesterol, and our blood levels decrease.

By keeping our carbohydrate consumption down, we can reduce our cholesterol in yet another manner. Cholesterol, as we discussed earlier, is made from a substance called acetyl-coenzyme A. Acetyl CoA is produced in several biochemical reactions in the body—mainly from the breakdown of fatty acids for energy—and then is used to make cholesterol and to feed into other biochemical processes. In the fasting state or in a diet low in carbohydrate, Acetyl CoA is shunted *away* from the cholesterol formation pathway and into the formation of ketones instead. So, when we consume few carbohydrates, we end up both decreasing the activity of the enzyme that regulates the rate of synthesis of cholesterol and reducing the availability of the substance from which cholesterol is made. These are the ways a low-carbohydrate diet reduces cholesterol levels, but our maintenance diet is more than just a low-carbohydrate diet.

Let's review the ways that our maintenance diet improves our blood lipid profile:

• reduces the synthesis of cholesterol by reducing the activity of the rate-limiting enzyme HMG CoA Reductase.

• reduces the synthesis of cholesterol by reducing the amount of Acetyl CoA available for conversion into cholesterol.

• soluble fiber prevents the reabsorption of cholesterol in the colon and increases its removal in the stool.

• soluble fiber blunts the blood sugar rise and subsequent insulin rise, therefore reducing cholesterol indirectly by reducing insulin levels.

• increased intake of monounsaturated fats brings about a lowering of cholesterol and LDL while at the same time increasing the amount of HDL.

• decreased intake of saturated fat that comes from avoiding the sugar-fat combination directly reduces cholesterol and LDL.

• EPA and GLA supplements, if taken, reduce cholesterol and LDL, and in some individuals increase HDL.

A Final Word About Insulin

We have spent most of this chapter discussing the effects of lower insulin levels on high blood pressure, carbohydrate metabolism, and elevated cholesterol levels, but insulin plays many other roles in regulating various other biochemical functions in our bodies. Since this is a book on weight loss, let's look at the way in which insulin helps regulate fat storage and fat breakdown.

Insulin increases the rate at which glucose is used by many of the body's tissues. Since this increased use of glucose occurs at the expense of fat use, when insulin levels are high, we don't break down fat and use it for energy. On the other hand, when insulin levels are kept low, we break down our fat stores—which we very much want to do on a weight-loss program—and use the released fatty acids for energy.

Increased insulin levels inhibit the action of the enzyme that actually breaks down the triglycerides in the fat cells and releases the fatty acids into the bloodstream where they are used for energy. At the same time, insulin increases the transport of glucose into the fat cells where it is then used to synthesize triglycerides. So, insulin tends to both increase the storage of fat and inhibit the breakdown of fat. These are two actions that we need to reverse on a regimen designed for losing fat.

When we keep our insulin levels low, as we do on the PSMF and the maintenance diet, our biochemistry favors the breakdown of fat and its use for energy. Low insulin levels mean a much more active enzyme that breaks down the contents of the fat cells and releases the fatty acids into the blood where they are transported to the tissues to be used for energy. Low insulin levels mean that much less glucose is transported into the fat cells, and therefore, fat storage is greatly diminished. In fact, when insulin isn't present in large enough amounts to facilitate this transport of glucose into the fat cells, fat storage is actually inhibited, even in the presence of considerable fat in the blood.

It should be apparent to you that you can do nothing but good for yourself by undertaking a regimen to stabilize your blood sugar and insulin levels. You will find that as you do, you will improve your health and at the same time reduce your stores of fat quickly. In my opinion, the PSMF followed by the maintenance diet is the best means we have available today to achieve this goal.

12

Nothing's Perfect

*O*N any sort of diet that you are likely to embark upon, you may have problems. These problems are generally minor and usually arise because you have changed your normal routine. Your body is used to the amount and type of food you have been feeding it, and it is likely to take notice when everything changes. The PSMF is a diet that is probably a great deal different from any that you may have been on (that's one of the reasons that makes it so effective), and it is apt to cause some of the little discomforts that you sense as your body adapts to a new way of eating. By the time you are on the maintenance diet, the low-carbohydrate way will all be old hat to your system, and you will suffer the discomfort only when you occasionally slip and revert to your old ways.

I don't want you to think, as you read the following list of problems, that you are going to get all, or even any, of them. Virtually all of my patients on the PSMF report that they feel better than they have in a long time. But almost everybody, at some point during their time on the PSMF, will have a bad day—and you probably will, too. You will just feel lousy; you won't necessarily be nauseated or have a headache or really anything specific, you'll just feel bad. I don't know why this happens, but it does. It is nothing you can't endure—just don't try to convince yourself that you need something to eat to bring you out of it. The feeling will be gone in a day.

The following list is not meant to take the place of a consultation with your doctor about any symptom that worries you. It is provided as a guideline for you to use in understanding and dealing with most of the minor symptoms you may encounter on the PSMF. It is the same list I give all my patients when they start the PSMF.

Headache

During the first few days on the diet, you may experience a headache that can range in severity from very mild to pretty painful. These headaches sometimes occur as you adapt to a lower blood sugar level and as you start to experience ketosis. They rarely last long and can be treated easily. As far as migraine headaches go, some patients have reported that their migraines diminished in severity or even vanished while on the PSMF; others have reported no change. I can't think of a patient who reported a migraine that worsened.

REMEDIES: A couple of Extra Strength Tylenol or the generic equivalent (500 mg of acetaminophen) should be all that is needed. Be very careful in taking aspirin or ibuprofen (Advil or Medipren) or any medication containing aspirin or ibuprofen. These medicines—or any anti-inflammatory medicines for that matter—can cause problems in the lining of the stomach, especially if taken without food as a buffer. If you are on prescription anti-inflammatory medicines for some reason, *always* take them with your meal or at the very least, with a supplement. Often, drinking a supplement, a diet drink, a cup of coffee, or a cup of bouillon will help resolve the headache. Any headache you might have that does not respond to these reasonable measures, and causes you significant discomfort, may be from causes other than the diet and should be discussed with your physician.

Dizziness

Because the PSMF is so effective in eliminating excess sodium and fluid from the body, you may be prone to a little dizziness or light-headedness in the early stages of the diet. This state occurs because your body fluid level drops more quickly than your circulatory system can adapt to the new, less-fluid-ridden you. This effect, which is most common in the summer, will be felt most noticeably when you change positions, for instance when standing up from a stooped, sitting, or lying posture, but it may also occur with just quiet standing or sitting for prolonged periods.

REMEDIES: First, make sure that you are indeed consuming at least 64 ounces of fluid daily. If you aren't, start; if you are, you can increase your fluid intake even more. The next step is to add a little salt to your diet to replace some of the lost sodium. You may do this by adding a little salt to your foods and supplements, by drinking a cup of bouillon, or by eating a dill pickle (dill pickles have almost no carbohydrate and are crawling with sodium). Have your blood pressure checked to be certain of your reading, especially if you were previously taking blood pressure medications or have a known history of problems related to blood pressure. If dizziness persists, consult your physician.

Constipation

Constipation seems to be perceived almost universally as a problem by dieters on the PSMF. I say "perceived" because it's more a problem of perception than an actual problem. People aren't really constipated, they just think they're constipated. It is perfectly normal while on the PSMF to have only two bowel movements per week. It stands to reason that if the PSMF is low in volume, and almost entirely used by the body, there is not much left to pass through. Don't worry about it. When you get on maintenance, your fiber intake will increase dramatically, and so will your bowel movement frequency. Some people are not willing, for whatever reason, to accept only two bowel movements per week—they feel compelled to move their bowels daily, whether they need to or not. And occasionally, some patients can have hard stools on the PSMF and irritate hemorrhoids or other rectal problems. Both of these groups of people can find relief by following the instructions given below.

REMEDIES: Add fiber to the diet. You may take FiberCon tablets (two of them 3 to 4 times a day with increased fluids), which have no taste but are relatively expensive; a less expensive alternative is Konsyl powdered fiber or the sugar-free form of Metamucil powder, both of which taste like cardboard in their natural state. You may mix these powdered fiber laxatives with sugar-free Tang or Crystal Light to make them more palatable, but DO NOT USE REAL ORANGE JUICE! All of these forms of fiber may be purchased without a prescription at groceries and drugstores. Stool softeners, such as Surfak (generic name: dioctyl sodium sulfosuccinate), taken as directed on the container, may also be of help. Another alternative to fiber or stool softeners is to take an enema periodically. Fleet effervescent enemas may be purchased at all supermarkets and drugstores. Serious constipation, especially if associated with nausea, vomiting, or cramping, should be evaluated by your physician right away.

Indigestion

This complaint is not frequent on a high protein diet, but if it does occur, it may be from too much acid/caffeine in the diet beverages, or too much coffee on an empty stomach.

REMEDIES: Decrease caffeine and carbonated-beverage intake by substituting water in supplements or using decaffeinated or non-carbonated liquids (decaf coffee/tea, Crystal Light, Kool-Aid, etc.). Most antacids are prepared with sugar, sorbitol, mannitol, or dextrose for flavor. Because all of these are carbohydrates and may interfere with the fat-burning process, they should be avoided. Try instead one tablespoon of baking soda dissolved in a glass of water as an antacid. If the indigestion causes severe discomfort, the diet may not be the cause. Consult your physician right away to be certain of the cause of the problem.

Leg or Foot Cramping

The level of potassium, an important electrolyte in the body, may become depleted on the PSMF, causing muscle cramping. This problem is often seen in the summer because of increased fluid loss through sweating, but it is not unusual in the winter when cold, damp weather makes muscle cramping more frequent on or off the diet. Cramps on the maintenance diet may also be a reflection of insufficient calcium, but on the PSMF, you should be getting enough from the milk in the supplements.

REMEDIES: If you suffer muscle cramping while on the PSMF, try increasing your intake of potassium by increasing the amount of NoSalt brand salt substitute (pure potassium) you are using. Your physician may prescribe some potassium supplements for you to take. If you are on the maintenance diet and cramping occurs, increase your consumption of cheese and milk products or purchase a calcium supplement. To preclude potassium deficiency, make more liberal use of NoSalt. Be certain, especially in summer, that you are taking in a sufficient amount of fluid. If cramping occurs in cold weather, you may also try putting the affected part into warm water and massaging it to relieve the cramp. Warming up slowly prior to exercising may help prevent cramping associated with your daily walk or other exercise regimen. If cramping still occurs, notify your physician, who will probably check your potassium levels and make the appropriate adjustments.

Nausea

As your body adapts to lower blood sugar, less food volume in the stomach, and ketones in the blood, you may incur some mild nausea. This will usually subside after a short time on the diet. Occasionally, drinking large volumes of very cold beverages may cause some nausea. I don't know why this is, but quite a few patients have reported it.

REMEDIES: Space your supplements out evenly so that you do not go for long periods without one. If you're mixing the shakes to an icy consistency, try using less ice, or even mixing them with hot water or coffee. If nausea is more severe, or a persistent problem, consult with your physician.

Hair Loss

Many stresses to the human body, such as a general anesthesia during surgery, a severe infection, a high fever, pregnancy, or a rigid diet, can cause the hair follicles to become dormant. When this happens, the hair stops growing. It doesn't fall out, it just stops growing. Some time later, usually two to three months, the hair follicles become active again. When they do become active, new hair starts to grow and pushes the old, dormant hair out. When this old hair starts to come out, the person shedding it notices it, usually with alarm. Actually, this indicates that a new, healthy growth of hair has started. We've rarely seen hair loss as much of a problem in our patients using the PSMF as presented in this book. But occasionally, some vitamin and/or mineral deficiencies can cause hair loss.

REMEDIES: If you are not taking the recommended amounts of vitamins and minerals, take them! If you are, and significant hair loss is occurring that is not being replaced by new, small hairs, consult your physician.

Menstrual Changes

With any major shift in metabolism, any significant loss of weight, or any substantial increase in activity level, the menstrual cycle may be affected. Some women experience a decrease in frequency, missed periods, or spotting; and others may experience just the reverse, with heavy flow for a longer period.

REMEDIES: If the changes are minor, don't be alarmed, unless of course you think you might be pregnant. (If you do think you may be pregnant, by all means get checked; if you are, you must stop the PSMF and discuss your diet with your obstetrician.) Your cycle will most likely return to normal during the course of the diet without any treatment at all. Be certain that you are taking the recommended amounts of vitamins, essential fatty acids, and minerals. If the symptoms are troublesome, the cramps severe, or the bleeding heavy, please consult your physician. If cramping is the primary symptom, again, be careful about taking ibuprofen or any medications containing aspirin because of the adverse effect these may have upon your stomach lining. Certainly these can be used if really needed, but with great care. There are also some medications your physician can prescribe that may help without risking harm to your stomach or to your diet.

Irritability

In the first few days of any diet, some patients notice an increase in irritability. The PSMF is no exception. There is a withdrawal period in dieting for several days that makes us grouchy. Again, this symptom is related to lowering blood sugar levels, to decreased food volume, and to adapting to ketosis. Don't despair if it happens to you, it will soon pass. In a few days, you will find yourself feeling more energetic and will most likely be filled with a sense of well-being.

REMEDIES: Time is the real remedy here, but until it passes, try sitting down to relax with a cup of bouillon, a diet drink, a cup of coffee, or a supplement. Get away from all hectic or noisy activity if possible and listen to some soothing music. You may find some relief in just closing your eyes for five minutes and letting your mind be blank. A gentle stroll at lunch, even in the middle of the afternoon if you can, may help.

Insomnia

Occasionally, I find patients to be sensitive to the increased amount of vitamin B_6 from the multivitamin they are taking. Large doses of this particular vitamin can cause insomnia. Heavy ketosis may also impair your ability to fall asleep.

REMEDY: If you are taking one of the recommended multi-vitamin supplements, you should have no problems as the amount of vitamin B_6 they contain is limited to the U.S. RDA. If you are taking another type of vitamin supplement, check the amount of vitamin B_6 in the formula. If it exceeds the U.S. RDA, switch to a different supplement that has a lower amount. You may notice that when you are in ketosis, taking your daily vitamins, and getting sufficient amounts of essential fatty acids, that you will require less sleep than you once did. This phenomenon should not be confused with insomnia. If you find yourself unable to get to sleep and stay asleep even though you are tired, then try adding a small amount of tryptophan (an amino-acid precursor of serotonin, the "sleep hormone," available at health food stores) with a cup of hot tea before bedtime. If insomnia persists, check your ketone level. If you are very strongly ketotic, you may need a slightly higher intake of carbohydrate. Try the changes we discussed in Chapter 6 to decrease your ketone levels slightly. If insomnia continues, consult your physician.

13

Exercise for
the Apathetic

*I*F you want to lose weight quickly, don't plan on losing it by exercising. Exercise has many benefits, but unfortunately, rapid weight loss is not one of them. Many people mistakenly believe that if they get out and walk or jog or swim or do aerobics, that they will miraculously lose their excess weight, and best of all, they will lose it without having to alter the way they eat. They enthusiastically throw themselves into some exercise regimen, then soon sadly realize that their efforts are not producing the desired results, become discouraged, and quit. To better understand how much time it takes to lose weight with exercise, let's look at some figures. If you start out jogging or walking for 35 miles each week—that's 5 miles per day, seven days per week—and you *don't* increase the amount of food you eat, you can plan on losing about one pound a week—or about 50 pounds in a year. Or you could go on the PSMF for 10 to 15 weeks and lose the same 50 pounds. In other words, you can lose the weight four or five times more quickly with dieting than you can with exercise. The quickest way of all to lose weight is with the combination of the PSMF *and* exercise.

Regular exercise of the right kind produces many improvements in health. It lowers total serum cholesterol, increases the HDL fraction of cholesterol, lowers serum triglyceride levels, lowers blood pressure, retards or prevents osteoporosis, improves glucose tolerance, decreases serum insulin levels, increases lean-body mass, decreases fat percentage, and reduces the risk of certain cancers. Exercise reverses or slows down many of the changes associated with aging, and in fact, by virtue of the reduction in risk for cardiovascular disease that it brings about, exercise actually contributes to longevity. In this chapter we will touch upon some of these benefits, but most of our time will be spent on the function of exercise as an aid to weight loss.

There are two types of exercise—isometric and isotonic. *Isometric exercise* is exercise done by exerting force against an immovable object or by slowly lifting heavy weights and doing few repetitions. The classic example of isometric exercise is weight lifting with heavy weights and few reps. This type of exercise increases strength and increases muscle mass, but it does little to enhance weight loss or to improve cardiovascular fitness. It does, however, have a place in an exercise regimen designed for our overall fitness, and we will discuss it in more detail later in the chapter.

Isotonic exercise is done by repetitive movements in which the muscle fibers are stretched and contracted without increasing the weight applied to them. Running, walking, swimming, bicycling— all are isotonic exercises. These exercises increase cardiovascular fitness and facilitate weight loss. Almost all exercise is a combination of isotonic and isometric exertion, with the activities commonly thought of as being endurance exercises being predominantly isotonic, and the strengthening or muscle-building workouts being mainly isometric. To eliminate confusion due to the similarity of the two words, from now on I will refer to isotonic exercise as endurance exercise and leave isometric as it is.

Exercise programs are similar to diets in that most people who start them don't stick with them for long. The reason? Like diets, most exercise programs are unpleasant and require us to deviate from the more familiar, comfortable, habitual course. Since the developers of the PSMF have created a rapid weight-loss regimen that is not unpleasant to stick with and the maintenance program previously discussed is easy to follow, the diet component of the diet and exercise equation has been made much easier. How about exercise, can it be made less unpleasant? Yes, it can. Exercise physiologists have developed a method that allows us to increase gradually our level of fitness without the usual early-phase burnout due to exhaustion. This method is called *pulse-driven exercise*. Before we examine this type of conditioning more closely, let's observe what happens to most people who start an exercise regimen.

I, like many people my age, got caught up in the jogging phenomenon. I had planned to spend about an hour per day running, but it turned out that it was more in the neighborhood of three hours. I would spend an hour dreading it, an hour actually jogging/walking, and another hour recovering. Needless to say, I didn't stick with my jogging plan for long. This, unfortunately, is the same path followed by many others. People typically have a perverse penchant for starting to exercise with much too much vigor. A session of overdoing it ends with the exerciser exhausted and sometimes even injured. The next day, or the one after that, he is invariably too sore to have much enthusiasm for continuing his program. This doesn't apply to everyone of course—some people continue until they get into shape and the exercise becomes enjoyable. Most, however, fall by the wayside. If you don't believe me, count the number of people you see jogging in your neighborhood on the first of January and compare it to the number you see on the first of June. This desertion from the ranks of those in the process of getting fit can be lessened by the use of pulse-driven exercise.

In order to better understand how the rigors of exercise can be made more tolerable early on, let's look at how your body responds to exertion by first noting the changes that you can observe—we'll discuss the chemical changes later. If, for example, you start to work out strenuously on an exercycle, you will find that with time your breathing becomes more and more labored until you reach the point at which you cannot continue. You will probably feel as if your legs could continue but not your lungs. Because of this dyspnea (difficult, almost painful, gasping for air) which lessens with improved fitness, most people assume that with progressive exercise their lung capacity is somehow improved. Several studies have shown that—assuming no disease—there is little difference in the lung capacity of a trained endurance athlete and that of a sedentary person of the same age. As we shall see, this dyspnea originates from chemical changes in the working muscles and not from inadequate lung capacity.

You will also notice during and immediately after vigorous exertion that your heart rate increases dramatically. The poorer your physical condition when you start exercising, the more quickly your heart rate increases and the longer it takes after exercise to return to normal. Conversely, as your level of conditioning improves, your heart rate will be slower when you are at rest, will not increase as quickly with exertion, and will return to normal much more quickly. Unlike the situation in the lungs, these changes do result in part from an improvement in the conditioning of the heart brought about by the exercise as well as from changes in the skeletal muscles being exercised. This ability to exercise longer without being winded and without having your heart pound is called the training effect, and it is brought about by regular endurance exercise. The best way of actually measuring this training effect or the change in fitness is by looking at changes in the maximal oxygen uptake brought about by a period of training.

The "maximal oxygen uptake" is defined as the largest amount of oxygen used by the body over a short period of time. It is a function of cardiac output—the amount of blood pumped by the heart—and muscle utilization—the amount of oxygen extracted by the muscles from the blood. With training, both the cardiac output and the muscle utilization of oxygen increase, bringing about an increase in the maximal oxygen uptake, which unfortunately must be measured in the laboratory. We will see later how to correlate this value with the heart rate so that you can measure your own improvement in fitness.

Two factors control cardiac output—heart rate and the amount of blood pumped with each heartbeat. For example, if your heart beats 70 times per minute and with each beat pumps about one-half cup of blood, then your cardiac output is 35 cups per minute. This 35 cups of blood being pumped every minute carries with it a specific amount of oxygen that can be released to the tissues. If the muscles require more oxygen—as they do during strenuous exercise—it can be provided by increasing the cardiac output and bringing more blood—and oxygen—to the muscles. Your heart can improve its output in two ways—by increasing its rate or by increasing the amount of blood pumped with each beat. By increasing your heart rate from 70 to 140 beats per minute, you will double your cardiac output and provide 70 cups per minute of blood to your muscles instead of 35. This is precisely what happens when you exercise vigorously—your heart rate rises to the occasion. Before you are conditioned, the only way your heart can increase the rate of blood flow to the muscles is by increasing its rate.

The second means your heart has to increase its output is by increasing the amount of blood discharged with each beat. If your heart increases the amount of blood pumped from one-half cup to one full cup per beat, then 70 cups per minute can be provided to the muscles while maintaining the rate at 70 beats per minute. In this example, the 35 cups of blood per minute required while the body is at rest can be maintained at a heart rate of only 35 beats per minute. This is the reason trained endurance athletes have heart rates in the neighborhood of 40 to 50 beats per minute—they have a much greater volume of blood expelled from their hearts with each beat. Progressive endurance exercise strengthens your heart by thickening the heart muscle so that it can eject the blood more forcefully and more completely with each contraction. The untrained or unconditioned heart doesn't completely empty with each contraction, but after a period of conditioning or heart-muscle strengthening, it does. The additional blood pumped with each stroke as the heart is conditioned provides more blood to the muscles without as great an increase in heart rate and is the basis for pulse-driven exercise. Before we examine this type of training more closely, let's look at what happens in the muscle tissue during exercise.

Muscles require energy to work. They require considerable energy for strenuous work, but they also require energy at rest and for nonstrenuous work. As I type this sentence, my arm, finger, and shoulder muscles are working—though at the speed I type, not strenuously—and require energy. The energy they use comes from three sources—free fatty acids (derived from fat tissue), glycogen (the storage form of glucose), and blood glucose itself. The relative amount of each of these three substances used for energy depends upon two factors: (1) the level of activity of the muscle, and (2) whether or not oxygen is present in the muscle. At low levels of exertion, the muscle favors the use of free fatty acids, but with increasing effort it tends to shift more to glycogen for energy, though still consuming some fat. As long as there is oxygen present, the muscle will continue to burn fat and glycogen as fuel. When the oxygen is entirely consumed, as it ultimately is during very strenuous exertion, the muscle shifts to the oxidation of glucose for energy, and no more fat and glycogen are used. In the absence of oxygen, the breakdown of glucose is inefficient, and the muscles soon cannot get enough energy and refuse to function. Usually before this happens and your muscles quit, you are out of breath. This dyspnea or shortness of breath also comes about because of the shift to the breakdown of glucose for energy that takes place when the muscle can't get enough oxygen to continue using fat and glycogen.

When your muscles break down glucose for energy with no oxygen present—or *an*aerobically—lactic acid is produced as a by-product. This lactic acid accumulates and would cause the blood to become acidic if it weren't for the buffering system we all have built into us. Your body buffers or neutralizes this excess lactic acid by combining it with other substances that result in its being broken down into molecules that the body can get rid of—among them carbon dioxide. You eliminate carbon dioxide by transporting it via the blood to your lungs, where it is removed as you exhale. As the lactic acid builds up as a result of anaerobic exercise and is buffered producing carbon dioxide, you must increase your respiratory rate to keep pace. In fact, your rate of respiration is driven involuntarily by the level of carbon dioxide in your blood and not by the level of oxygen present. You have receptors located in your neck and in other parts of your body that monitor the level of carbon dioxide in your blood, and via nerves that feed back through the brainstem, they cause you to breathe when that level reaches a certain point. If you hold your breath for as long as you can, the overwhelming urge to breathe that you finally give in to comes not from a lack of oxygen, but from the increase in carbon dioxide in your blood. When your muscles produce carbon dioxide from the anaerobic use of glucose for energy, you feel this same shortness of breath or dyspnea. It is this increase in carbon dioxide production that causes you to feel winded after strenuous exercise, and that causes you finally to quit—not the fact that your lungs are not in shape.

What does all this tell us about weight loss and pulse-driven exercise? It tells us that if we do endurance types of exercise starting at low levels of intensity and progressing, as measured by our heart rate, we will not only not be tired, sore, and miserable, but we will actually break down fat and build muscle more quickly. The most rapid way we can increase the oxygen delivered to our muscles is to increase our heart rate. Muscle tissue needs oxygen to break down fat efficiently and use it as an energy source. The harder the muscle works, the more oxygen it needs, and consequently the faster the heart beats to provide the oxygen. As soon as the muscle can't get enough oxygen because it is working too strenuously, it shifts to glucose for fuel and no more fat is broken down. Since we want fat to be broken down, we want to keep the muscle working at a low enough intensity that it always has enough oxygen to continue to use fat for fuel. We have no way of actually monitoring the level of oxygen in the tissues, but we can monitor our heart rate. During exertion, as long as our heart rate doesn't exceed a certain threshold, we can be assured that our muscles are getting adequate oxygen to continue consuming fat and are said to be undergoing "aerobic" exercise.

The use of the word "aerobic" compels me to digress. "Aerobic" must have been one of those words Lewis Carroll had in mind when he had Humpty-Dumpty say to Alice: "When I make a word do a lot of work like that, I always pay it extra." "Aerobic" is a well-paid word indeed. We have "low-impact aerobics" and logically, "high-impact aerobics," "aerobic dancing," "rhythmic aerobics," "water aerobics," aerobics this and aerobics that *ad nauseam*. The word "aerobics" by itself conjures up visions of an attractive, very slender, young lady dressed in leotards, gyrating and rhythmically flailing each appendage to the beat of some torchy rock song—while the students, most of whom are older and out of shape, desperately try to keep pace. "Aerobics" simply means that the muscles are exercising in the presence of oxygen and are using fat and glycogen for fuel. People truly doing "aerobics" are working at a level of mild exertion, as determined by their heart rate, that keeps them from being out of breath and keeps their muscles consuming fat and glycogen. In the scene described above, the young lady is doing "aerobics," but most of the people in the class are not. Don't set your rate of exercise to keep pace with someone else—keep pace by monitoring your own heart rate.

As we age, the maximal heart rate we can achieve decreases, and as a rule of thumb, it can be calculated by subtracting our age from 220. For example, if you are forty, then your maximal heart rate would be estimated as 180 beats per minute (220 minus 40). If you have been sedentary for some time and wish to start an exercise program, you should start out by exercising at a level of intensity that will increase your heart rate to 65 percent of maximal—in the case of the forty-year-old above, around 115 to 120 beats per minute. The more overweight and out of shape you are, the higher your resting heart rate will be, and the less exertion will be required to raise your heart rate to 65 percent of maximal. If you are forty years old and are sixty pounds overweight, your resting heart rate may be 100 beats per minute, and it may take very little exertion to raise the rate to 120. Don't worry, that is exactly what you want to do—very little exertion. You want to keep your muscles working aerobically, and if you overexert you will be exercising anaerobically, huffing and puffing, and being miserable.

With time, as you continue to exercise aerobically, your heart will strengthen and each beat will become more forceful, expelling more blood to your muscles. Since each beat expels more blood, your resting heart rate will decrease as your heart strengthens, and more exertion will be required to elevate to the 120-beat-per-minute level. Although you will be working harder, you won't feel as if you are exerting yourself more than you did when you first started, and you will be customizing your aerobic workout to your own physiology.

The easiest way to monitor your pulse rate is to check your carotid pulse. This is the pulse in your carotid arteries, which are located on both sides of your neck. Gently feel around on either side of your Adam's apple with your index and second finger until you find your pulse. If you have trouble finding it, ask your physician or nurse to point it out for you. During your exercise, you should periodically stop and check your pulse to make sure that it is in the right range. Check it for six seconds, then multiply the number of beats you counted by ten. If during a brisk walk you count 12 beats in 6 seconds, your pulse would be 10 times that, or 120 beats per minute. If that is where it should be, great. If it is too high, then you should slow your walk down a little, or if it is too low, you should walk faster.

You should increase your pulse rate to 65 percent of maximal during each workout for the first month, then you should increase it to 70 percent of maximal. Maintain it at this higher rate for the next month, and then at the start of the third month increase it to 80 percent of your maximal heart rate. By the end of the third month, you will really be getting a workout, but if you have been faithful, it won't seem any more strenuous than it did when you began. This one-month, two-month, three-month, 65-, 70-, 80-percent progression is not chiseled into stone—if you feel as if you are over-exerting and are out of breath, take it more slowly. To get optimal benefit from aerobic exercise, you should do it at least three times per week, preferably five, and during each session you should keep your pulse rate up to the appropriate percentage of maximal for at least twenty minutes.

All this business about pulse taking and percent maximal heart rate may sound like a hassle, and you may be thinking that you don't really want to get involved with all that. I'm not going to let you get away that easily. There is a simple, hassle-free method of aerobic monitoring. You simply walk or jog at a rate that is brisk but allows you to carry on a conversation. This means talking—not gasping out words between breaths. If you have no exercise partner, talk to yourself, or if this seems less than dignified, sing. As your conditioning improves, you will be able to walk or jog much faster while still conversing.

If you're not going to buy the talking or singing method of pulse monitoring, you can simplify it even further. There is no reason— other than sloth—that you cannot undertake the following method. If sloth it be—see Chapter 14. Other than a body that is capable of walking, the only two pieces of equipment you will need are a watch and one eye. This method involves walking a distance that you measure, but doing it a little differently. Before we discuss it, let's look at the way many others start a similar program.

When most people start a walking or running program, they lay out a course that they intend to cover. It might be twice around the block or to a particular cross-street or other landmark and back. They then record the amount of time it takes them to walk or jog this distance, and then they try to decrease this time on each successive loop around the course. This is the wrong way to go about it.

To get the maximum benefit from walking or running, you should progressively increase your expenditure of energy. To do this, first determine how much time you intend to devote to this activity each time you undertake it. If, for instance, you plan on spending thirty minutes per day walking, and plan on doing this five days per week, you should start by walking fifteen minutes in a direction away from home, make note of the distance you covered, then walk the fifteen minutes back home. Next, each day, try to increase the distance that you walk while sticking to your thirty-minute time limit. If you follow this program for several months, you will be in condition without once having had to count your pulse or sing to yourself.

The reason this method works so well is that it forces you to expend a little more energy each day that you exercise, just as monitoring your pulse does. Most people don't realize that they expend the same amount of energy in casually strolling along for one mile that they do in running the same one mile full out. It doesn't seem reasonable, but it is. It takes the same amount of energy to move your body over a given course irrespective of how fast you move it. Granted, you get a little conditioning by trying to decrease your time around a certain distance, but you don't increase your energy expenditure. So, gradually increase your distance, and the rest will take care of itself.

Let's summarize the advantages of endurance or isotonic exercise. With time and progressive fitness you will strengthen your heart, increase your lean-body mass, decrease your fat mass, decrease your cholesterol, increase your HDL, make yourself less susceptible to osteoporosis, strengthen your tendons and ligaments, increase the circulation to your muscles, decrease your blood pressure, and *lose weight*. The foregoing are all things that can be measured, but many unmeasurable or subjective factors will be improved. You will feel better, you will be more energetic, and you will be more alert and adept at dealing with day-to-day life. If you are physically able, start an endurance exercise program now.

Isometric Exercise

We've seen the way in which endurance exercise helps us lose weight, but what about isometrics? Isometric exercise doesn't actually help you lose weight—in fact, if you undertake a strenuous program of weight lifting, you may gain weight. But isometrics do make an important contribution to your total exercise program. Studies are appearing that indicate that a mild course of weight lifting is beneficial to people of all ages—even the elderly. Although they don't provide all the cardiovascular benefits that endurance programs do, weight-lifting regimens increase HDL (although not as much as endurance exercise), increase bone density (retard or even reverse osteoporosis), increase lean-body mass, and strengthen tendons, ligaments, and muscles, making them much less prone to injury. As with endurance exercises, there are several ways of doing isometrics, ranging from the good to the dangerous. Let's look at a method that is fun and easy, yet will increase your strength and power quickly.

The title of this chapter—written tongue firmly in cheek—is meant to imply that the exercise programs discussed are not designed to develop world-class athletes, but to show how to undertake a conditioning program that is fun and effective, yet not exhausting or injurious. As is the case with endurance regimens, isometric regimens have the potential for damage both to your morale and to your body if not done properly, or if tackled too aggressively early on. An illustration of the improper way to start a program of weight training is provided by my favorite bad example—me.

A few years ago, I went skiing for a week. I hadn't really skied much since college, and so I was ill prepared for the rigors of the slopes—not to mention the thin mountain air. After the first day, I could barely walk. I hurt everywhere, but especially in my legs, and after two days I developed an effusion (joint fluid accumulation) in my left knee. I determined that prior to the next year's ski season, I would join a gym and start weight training to better develop the muscles in my legs and to strengthen the ligaments around my knees. The next year, a month before ski season, I joined a gym. I had always thought that I had a reasonably decent-looking physique until my first workout. The weight room was swarming with massive, heavily muscled people who made me look puny by comparison, and the air was buzzing with excited conversation in which words such as "bulking," "definition," " 'roids," "lats," "abs," and "reps" were being thrown about. There were people who were actually screaming out as they tried to lift huge amounts of weight—it looked like the place for me. If I couldn't get in shape there, I couldn't get in shape. My conditioning "counselor" resembled the Hulk, but he was very solicitous as he explained how all the equipment worked and set out a course of exercise that would get me into shape for skiing. I started out on my regimen using light weights and working slowly and smoothly, and feeling pretty good about the whole thing until I noticed the Hulk eyeing me menacingly. Finally, he walked over to where I was lying on my back and lifting weights with my legs.

"You need more weight," he said. "You'll never get in shape unless you work harder." He added some weight to the machine.

"I don't really want to hurt myself," I said. "Since this is my first time, I just want to do a light workout."

"There's no such thing as a light workout—you can either play or you can work out; if you're going to work out you need to work."

"My legs are starting to hurt—and even my back," I said as I continued to lift.

"Give me just five more reps."

"My doctor told me not to do anything that would hurt my back," I lied in desperation.

"This'll make your back stronger—just two more."

"I can't do the last one, my legs hurt too much."

"Come on, you can do it." Then he finally said it: "NO PAIN, NO GAIN."

From the grunts, groans, and yelling I was hearing, I figured that people must be gaining all over the place, so with a grunt of my own I struggled through my last "rep." The Hulk then told me that we would concentrate on the lower body only—thank God—during this workout, and he proceeded to lead me through the rest of the machines until my legs were spaghetti.

"We'll hit the upper body next time," he said, waving as I staggered out.

Do you think I went back? Actually I did, but I made sure to go at a time when the Hulk wasn't there. By the time I ran into him again, he had found new meat and left me alone.

The point of all that is that *you*, not someone else, should control your workout. "No pain, no gain" is absolute nonsense. If it hurts, you are lifting incorrectly and risk injuring your back. Don't let your competitive nature goad you into overdoing it—you will accomplish much more, and do it comfortably (less pain, more gain?), if you do isometric exercise according to the instructions that follow.

In trying to develop yourself through weight training, you want to increase both strength and power. Strength is the ability of a muscle to contract against a given load. If you can press 200 pounds above your head, you have strength. Power—strength divided by time—is a much better indicator of athletic ability than is strength alone, and it is defined as the speed with which a muscle can contract under a given load. The more rapidly a muscle can contract against an opposing force, the more power it has. Pressing the 200 pounds above your head slowly shows that you have strength; snapping it up quickly demonstrates power. A good golf swing, skiing, basketball, tennis, racquetball, squash, crew—all these sports, and many others, require power to a much greater extent than they do strength. Power—not strength—is what allows you to move quickly and forcefully in an emergency situation, be it self-defense or self-preservation. The method of training with weights that I am about to describe will develop power in your muscles as well as strength.

As far as I am concerned, there are five cardinal rules of weight training that should always be followed in order to make rapid progress and prevent injury:

1. Always do the exercise with proper form.
2. Increase speed first, then weight
3. Never strain
4. Breathe normally while working out—don't hold your breath
5. Never, never arch your back while lifting weights.

To apply these rules to a specific exercise, let's look at the bench press. You do a bench press while lying on your back on a narrow bench holding the weight bar with your hands slightly wider than your shoulders. You extend your arms, forcing the weight bar upward, then you allow the bar to come back to almost touching your chest, then push it up again. You do a certain number of repetitions or "reps" of this exercise, rest for a time, then do another "set" of "reps." If you ever watch people do this exercise in a gym, you will notice that they have pretty good form for the first several reps, or maybe even the first set or two, but ultimately they start to strain, hold their breath, arch their backs, and struggle slowly to push the bar up. It looks like great fun, doesn't it? You don't want to follow their example.

Start out by keeping the weight light enough so that you can do three sets of ten reps each without having to strain. Don't worry if everyone else is lifting more than you are, you will catch up. At each exercise session, and I recommend no more than three per week, try to do each set a little more quickly. When you reach the point where you are doing the exercise, in this case the bench press, rapidly—it is time to go up on the weight. Add an amount of weight to the bar that will allow you to do your three sets, but more slowly—still without straining. If at any time you are arching your back or holding your breath to get the last few reps up, you are lifting too much weight. By pursuing this relatively relaxed regimen, you will be developing power in your muscles as well as strength. You will notice a difference in your golf game and in any other physical activities you enjoy.

It is beyond the scope of this book to detail all the various types of weight lifting exercises commonly done, but there are any number of good books available that demonstrate proper form. All exercises are not equal—in fact some are very risky. A good book on muscle conditioning with examples of all the weight-related and stretching exercises you should avoid is *The Rejuvenation Strategy* by Rene Cailliet, M.D., and Leonard Gross. I highly recommend this book—you should read it before you begin any exercise program.

Spot Reducing

Only one thing can be said about spot reducing: in the absence of liposuction it can't be done—*except* in the abdominal area. Fat can't be preferentially removed from the waistline, but the waistline can become smaller. All it takes is attention to posture. If you stand up straight and pull in your belly, it will make an incredible difference in your appearance, while at the same time putting your spine in the position it was meant to be in. Don't slouch.

You can help your posture and your waistline by exercising specifically to strengthen your abdominal musculature. The best exercise for this is not the sit-up, but the sit-back. Abdominal muscles are not dynamic muscles—they don't routinely contract as do leg or arm muscles. They statically hold your abdominal contents in place. Most people who are overweight have lax abdominal muscles, and when these muscles are strengthened, their waistlines become much smaller, even in the absence of weight loss.

You perform the sit-back by sitting on the floor with your back straight up and your knees bent, hooking your feet under something or having someone hold them, and with your hands clasped behind your neck, start bending back at the waist until your stomach muscles feel tight. Try to hold this position for a count of twenty. If you can't, move your hands from behind your neck and cross them in front of your chest. Keep moving your crossed arms lower in front of you until you can do the sit-back for a count of twenty. Keep working until you can do it five times for a count of twenty each time, then start increasing the resistance by moving your hands higher and higher. Don't strain, and don't try to progress too quickly. This is a wonderful exercise that will improve the tone of your abdomen better than anything else I know.

Exercise Maintenance

Just as in weight maintenance, exercise maintenance is something you must do as long as you want to be fit. If you go back to your old way of eating, you will regain your weight; if you quit exercising, you will lose your level of fitness. Fortunately, exercise —after you are fit—will feed upon itself, and you will want to continue it because it's fun. But as with the dieting maintenance plan, you can take short vacations and indulge yourself in sloth. Just remember to monitor your pulse when you start back and reduce your level of exertion to correspond to the level of fitness you've dropped back to—keep it easy and aerobic. As long as you watch your pulse, you won't overexert.

A pulse-driven endurance exercise program coupled with an isometric regimen as detailed above will keep you in excellent physical condition—without causing you to dread doing it. You will stay lean, firm, and energetic without being sore, tired, and injured. Best of all, most of the diseases and "normal" progressions of aging will be staved off longer, and your body will actually become more youthful. If exercise can keep you healthy, youthful, less prone to injury, and feeling terrific—and it can, if done as described—then start today.

14

Discipline as
an Art Form

*N*OT long ago, an old college friend of mine traveling through town paid me a visit. He came with his wife, who is afflicted with AIDS—a tragic, invariably terminal disease, which she contracted from a blood transfusion some years before. My friend —a petroleum engineer—lives in Houston and designs refineries for one of the major oil companies. Over the past several years, the petroleum industry has suffered an economic downturn resulting in many layoffs, staff transfers, and consolidations. My friend, by virtue of his ability and length of employment, had been able to avoid most of the upheaval, but unfortunately it finally caught up with him. He was transferred from his department and put on leave of absence until his new position—one he didn't want—was opened. He took the several weeks available and spent them traveling with his wife, and thus his visit to me.

The last time I had seen Jack, six or so years before, he was starting to develop a little "middle-age spread," and I expected him to be heavier yet. I was very surprised when I opened the door and found him looking trim and fit. Later, during dinner at one of my favorite restaurants, one that specializes in fabulous dessert concoctions—I had taken a little dietary vacation in honor of their visit—he ate a steak and a salad and couldn't be persuaded even to nibble on anything from the pastry cart. He had coffee while the rest of us ploughed into some delicious gooey dessert that we all later regretted having eaten. Knowing his predilection for sweets in the past (he lived on them in college), I asked him why the change. His response—the reasoned reaction from a very rational mind—caused me to change my thinking on the whole idea of eating.

"Mike, my life is in enormous turmoil. My wife is sick with a disease that I can't understand, and can't do anything about. My job has been in jeopardy, and now I've been moved—against my will—to a position that I don't want, and probably can't perform very well. I had no choice—it was either change or resign, and with Nancy's illness, I couldn't afford to be without insurance, so even my option to resign was taken away. I'm being bounced along by events over which I have no control whatsoever—I can't control this disease and I can't control what happens to me at work, in fact, I don't even know how long I'll be in this new position, or if I'll even be working beyond that. At this point, my diet, my weight, and my physical condition are a few of the only things left in my life that I *can* control—and I intend to control them. That's why I watch my diet and don't eat sweets."

Prompted by my friend's eloquent, well-reasoned response, I began to think very seriously about this business of control over eating. Most people have the reverse of the problem Jack had—they are in control of most aspects of their lives but are completely out of control when it comes to their eating. I don't know how many people I've seen who are professionals of one sort or another—executives, politicians, or even career military officers—and who overeat and are overweight. These are people who hold demanding positions requiring considerable self-discipline and sac-rifice. They don't hesitate to throw themselves fully into projects that entail monumental sacrifices of their time and energy; they are exacting people who demand near perfection in themselves and others; yet they are unable to control their own eating. Mainly, I think, because they, unlike my friend Jack, don't look upon eating as something that—like other facets of their lives—is subject to their control. But it is.

There are many circumstances over which we have no control whatsoever. The weather, the economy, the actions of our cowork-ers, the misdeeds of elected officials, the misbehavior of grown children—all these things, and many like them, we have little con-trol over, yet we find ourselves worrying about them, considering all sorts of options to change somehow the behaviors of other people or to modify affairs that we have no power to modify. (I'm not saying that we can't insulate ourselves from changes in the economy, inclement weather, actions of other people, etc., because we can, we just can't change those things themselves.) We waste who knows how much time and emotional energy in trying to change situations that we can't change, yet *we often refuse to change the situations over which we have complete control.* Let's look at a couple of examples.

My wife and I had been friends for several years with a couple I will call George and Elizabeth. They had been married for almost twenty-five years and were seemingly very happy when George precipitately announced that he wanted a divorce. Elizabeth was devastated and was willing to do practically anything to keep their marriage together; she begged, she wept constantly, she threatened suicide, she promised to change, but through it all George remained resolute. He moved out, contacted an attorney, and filed for divorce. All the nightmarish workings of the divorce process began, and Elizabeth was finally left with a reasonable settlement, but without the person with whom she had spent the last twenty-five years of her life.

Soon after the divorce was final, George was dating a woman about fifteen years his junior whom he quickly married. He found a new job and moved with his new wife to another state. Elizabeth had been devastated by the divorce, but she was almost destroyed by this latest development. My wife and I and our friends did everything we could to help Elizabeth. We counseled her, we tried to introduce her to new people, we took her out with us, we listened to her endless analyses of why and how her marriage had failed and what she should have done about it—in short, we did everything imaginable to ease her grief, but without much success. She spent every waking hour absorbed in thoughts of George and what she could do to bring about a reconciliation, and she was still doing so two years after her divorce. It was obvious that there would be no reconciliation, but still she forged on.

Her constant ruminating on George caused Elizabeth to perform poorly at her job as a clothing buyer at a large department store, and she was finally demoted to a less demanding position. Her friends tired of hearing about George's latest treachery and began to visit less and less frequently. Even her children—the youngest was in college at the time of the divorce—were miserable in her company and made their visits shorter and less frequent. In fact, the children spent more time with George and their new stepmother—a situation that increased Elizabeth's burden.

By spending all her energies being obsessed with George's defection and remarriage, a circumstance over which she had absolutely no control, Elizabeth became a poor employee, an unwelcome neighbor, a person to be avoided, and a much less effective parent. She *could* control her eating, but she didn't; she first lost weight, then turned to food for solace and gained over fifty pounds. She *could* control her appearance, but she didn't; having a job in the fashion industry, she had always dressed stylishly, but she began to be increasingly slovenly. She *could* control her conversation, but she didn't; by constantly talking of George, she finally drove most of her friends away. Prior to her divorce, she was bright, capable, articulate, attractive, and industrious; after the divorce, all changed as she sank into a morass of self-pity.

The point of this story is that Elizabeth chose to be unhappy, perpetuating her unhappiness by refusing to take control of her life. By refusing to control those things she could, and by instead spending her life trying to control something she couldn't—George's behavior—she was destined for an existence of unending misery. Fortunately, Elizabeth's story has a happy ending, although it was several years in coming. She finally—at the urging of all who stuck by her—went to an excellent therapist who was able to convince her that there was life after George, but not without her willingness to meet the challenge. She took control of her life and is now remarried and happier than she was before her divorce. Ironically, George, whom I had occasion to talk with recently, wistfully mentioned that perhaps he had made a mistake—apparently, he is not entirely happy with his new bride.

Richard W., a patient of mine, was another example of someone whose life was careening out of control. He first came to see me—at his wife's insistence—for a complete physical examination. He was forty-eight years old, about forty-five pounds overweight, smoked two to three packs of cigarettes per day, never exercised, had a stressful job and a strong family history of heart disease—his father had died of a heart attack at age fifty-two. If there was ever a coronary disaster waiting to happen, it was Richard. On physical exam, I found him to have only mildly elevated blood pressure, a normal EKG, but very high serum cholesterol. In spite of his lack of severe high blood pressure and his normal EKG, he was clearly headed for serious trouble.

I presented the facts to Richard. I told him that he had every cardiac risk factor known to man, and that he was probably living on borrowed time. I told him that although he couldn't change his family history, he could make an effort to eliminate his other risks. I told him first that he needed to lose weight.

"I'd like to, and I've tried, I really have. My wife is always putting me on some kind of diet, but I go out with clients and I can't diet in front of them. Whenever I don't eat, I get very nervous—I don't think I could ever really diet."

"What about your smoking? You should quit," I told him.

"I've tried, I really have. I quit once for almost a week, and it about killed me. It's kind of like the dieting bit—every time I try to quit, I get so nervous that I can't even concentrate. I feel like I put more stress on my heart by trying to quit than by just going ahead and smoking."

"How about exercise?" I asked, but I knew the answer.

"I really don't have the time, with work and all. I tried to jog once and I was sore for a week—I even missed a day of work, and I can't miss work."

And so it went. I questioned Richard about the stress level of his job. He told me that his job was stressful, but that he enjoyed it. He said that the pressure from his job was stress he thrived on, not like the stress "caused by the kid." The "kid," it turned out, was Richard's only child, a twenty-six-year-old son who had dropped out of school, was living with his girlfriend, was unemployed, and was probably "doing dope." Richard talked with more animation and emotion about this wayward son than about any other topic. He had tried to provide for his son, he had "given him everything," he had "slaved and worked so that the kid could have a good education," and he was devastated by his son's ruinous behavior. This son, I learned, had been leading this dissolute life for the past *five* years.

Richard, like Elizabeth, was investing huge amounts of emotional energy in a situation over which he had no control. His son was—from whatever sources—self-supporting, and he was not about to yield to parental pressure. Richard had "cut him off" financially but could bring no other pressure to bear. I tried to convince him that this son, at twenty-six years old, was no longer his father's responsibility, but I wasn't successful.

I told Richard that he needed to see a cardiologist and get a stress test, that he should lose weight, stop smoking, and after he saw the cardiologist, start some light exercise. His response was that he couldn't do any of these things until "this kid business is all straightened out."

Eleven months later, Richard had a heart attack. It happened during one of his son's infrequent visits home, in the course of a harsh argument over "taking responsibility." Fortunately, Richard was taken quickly to the hospital and he survived without much permanent heart muscle damage.

I have never had a heart attack, but I have taken care of many who have. Most victims say that the chest pain is crushing and of extreme intensity. They can't get enough air, they perspire profusely, and they uniformly believe that death is imminent. Richard had all these symptoms, and this glimpse of his own mortality and subsequent hospital stay changed him immeasurably.

He quit smoking, and under the guidance of his cardiologist, he started a progressive walking regimen. He lost weight. During his hospitalization, he established a sort of reconciliation with his son. He is back at work and feels better than he has in years. He still occasionally becomes angry over his son's style of living—which hasn't changed—but he is now able to recognize that his son is beyond his control. Richard now channels this anger into productive forms where it is harmlessly dissipated.

Richard found that he could quit smoking, he could diet, he did have time for exercise—he had control over his behavior. The reason he took this control was that he desired to continue living, and without the changes that taking control brought about, he wasn't likely to continue living for long. Although he doesn't have control over his son and realizes that he never will, he has slowly quit worrying about it. He is on the road to a much better life.

Why am I discussing these cases in a diet book? Neither Elizabeth nor Richard ever went on the diet described here. Why do their cases matter? Their cases matter because they demonstrate how normal, bright, hardworking people can refuse to take control over very controllable aspects of their lives, while at the same time becoming overwhelmed by events that are uncontrollable. Contrast their cases with my friend Jack's. Jack was burdened with incredible adversity over which he had no control, but he seized control over that which he could—his diet and his fitness. He controls what he can, and as a result, he is better equipped physically and mentally to deal with the circumstances that he can't control. If he had reacted to stress in the same manner as did our other examples, his physical condition would have deteriorated and he would probably have been on the road to mental illness as well. All these cases are extreme, but they demonstrate that even in extraordinary situations control can be achieved: either early, as in Jack's case, or later, after disastrous consequences, as with Richard and Elizabeth.

You may not be able to control anything else, but you can control your eating. The PSMF requires some discipline and control, especially in the first few days before hunger disappears. The maintenance diet requires little discipline—but it does require some. You must recognize that you have complete control over your progress on this diet. If you seize control and follow the dietary guidelines, you will be successful; if you don't, you won't.

You should regard your diet and your new slimmer figure as you would anything else requiring effort to maintain. You wouldn't work diligently and sacrifice your time and energy to obtain a better job only to slack off, loaf, and get fired after reaching your goal. Why do it with your diet? When you were in school, you didn't stay up late with your nose in a book and sacrifice your weekends studying to do well on an exam, only to give a halfhearted effort and blow it. Why do it with your diet? If you have reached adulthood, gone to school, and maintained a job, you have exercised discipline. You may have exercised more or less discipline than others, but you have exercised discipline nevertheless. And discipline, like any other skill, becomes more proficient with use. Use it.

If circumstances arise that burden you emotionally, don't bolt from your diet and seek comfort in food. Analyze the situation and determine whether or not you can do anything about it. If you can, take the appropriate action; if not, recognize the fact and try to focus your energies elsewhere. You will always have control of your diet. Don't relinquish it. An excellent book on control is *Take Effective Control of Your Life* by William Glasser, M.D. Even if you are living a problem-free life, this book will help you, but if you are in a situation similar to Richard's, Elizabeth's, or Jack's, you will profit enormously from it.

Dr. Glasser says, basically, that there are four components to any behavior: the doing component, the feeling component, the thinking component, and the physiological component. Of the four, we have complete control only over the doing component, and partial control over the thinking component—over the other two, we have no control whatsoever. Dr. Glasser touches on diet only peripherally in his book, so let's look at how these components and our control over them apply to eating.

If we haven't eaten for a time and we see or smell food that appeals to us, we feel hungry—the feeling component. We can't help it that we feel hungry, it's beyond our control. Our mouths water and our stomachs growl—the physiological component. We can't keep our salivary glands from working, and we can't do anything about our intestinal muscles that are becoming active. We have no control over these physiological processes. We look at the food and smell the aroma, and we imagine how good it will taste —the thinking component. As long as we are hungry and in the presence of this wonderful food, we will probably think about it. We can, however, force ourselves to think of other things, but more than likely, our thoughts will occasionally revert back to the food. We can partially control our thinking—the stronger-willed of us more than others. We sit down and eat the food—the doing component. This act, we can completely control. We can eat or not, as we please. Unlike the workings of our salivary glands, or our feelings of hunger, we have total, 100-percent control over whether or not we eat.

The interesting thing about all this is that although many of us allow the uncontrollable components of behavior to direct the controllable component, it can work in the reverse direction. If we take charge of the doing component, over which we have total control, the other involuntary components will fall into step. In our example above, if we walk away from the food and involve ourselves in a different activity, one unrelated to food or eating, slowly our feelings, physiology, and thinking will change and adapt themselves to our new activity. We have controlled what we can and as a result, have ended up controlling indirectly those components that we can't control directly.

If you are now, or have ever been, overweight, you have let the components of behavior over which you have no control coerce your doing or controllable component into submission. You have been confronted with greasy, carbohydrate-laden, unhealthful, but unfortunately, very tasty foods, and you have let the feeling and physiological components of behavior bias your thinking component. Then all three put your doing component to the sword, and you ate that which in your heart you knew you shouldn't. If you were like most victims, you probably said that you "couldn't help it.'' But you could, and you can now. Take charge of your actions —you have total control of them. Everything else will fall in line.

Unlike your prehistoric ancestors, who had external controls on their diet—they could only eat what they worked hard to obtain—you must be willing to put internal controls in place to lose weight successfully. By adhering to the PSMF, you will lose weight and reach your goal—but only if you maintain control of your actions and refuse to succumb to the many involuntary feelings and physiological urgings you may experience. The diet was designed to minimize hunger, but occasionally you will need to use your powers of control to achieve your goal. On the maintenance portion of the program, you will be able to indulge your feelings and physiology to a much greater extent, but you must realize that you cannot go back to your previous way of eating—unless you want to go back to your previous weight. Your genetic makeup is such that you must diet to maintain your weight, and this maintenance diet allows you more latitude than any other I know of. In spite of this greater latitude, you will still need to control the doing component of your behavior to achieve successful maintenance.

If you have a moment of weakness, all is not lost. If you are on the PSMF component when this happens, just continue on with your supplements. If on maintenance, spend a couple of days on the recovery diet. Just DO NOT give up completely. If you find yourself losing your willpower, reread this chapter. Profit from the experiences of Richard and Elizabeth and don't refuse to take control. YOU *CAN* TAKE CONTROL, BUT *YOU* MUST DO IT.

Good Luck

APPENDIX A

How to Find a Doctor

The most obvious choice for a physician is your own family doctor. He or she knows you well and is in the best position to judge whether or not you are suited for the PSMF. Your family physician may decide to monitor you on the program or may elect to refer you to a specialist in bariatrics —the specialty of medicine that deals with the treatment of weight problems and diseases associated with obesity.

If you have no family physician, your best bet is to check in the telephone directory under "Physicians/bariatrics." If there is no listing there, look under "Weight Control Services." You will find all manner of different weight-reduction centers in this section, but look for a center that is affiliated with a physician. Be careful—many centers give the appearance of having a physician on their staff when actually they don't. Make sure that you see a doctor in an office setting—not a weight-loss center that may have a physician merely drop by to give you a physical and then never be seen again. Make sure the physician is available for consultation throughout the program.

To insure that you get a physician who specializes in the treatment of people with weight problems, you may call or write:

American Society of Bariatric Physicians
5600 S. Quebec Street, Suite 160D
Englewood, Colorado 80111
Phone: 1-303-779-4833

This group will give you the name, address, and telephone number of a bariatric physician in your area.

You may also write or call the protein supplement manufacturers listed below. Representatives of these companies will be very happy to direct you to a physician in your area who uses their supplements and follows patients on the protein-sparing fast.

LifePlus
Benn Kel Corporation
Nutritional Products Division
P.O. Box 1179
Sparks, MD 21152-9981
Phone: 1-800-541-3121

R-kane Products, Inc.
8351 National Highway
Pennsauken, NJ 08110
Phone: 1-800-237-9765

Robard Corporation
Medical Nutritional Systems Division
821 East Gate Drive
Mt. Laurel, NJ 08054
Phone: 1-800-222-9201

Mail-Order Sources and Product Information

Protein Supplement Powders

Almost every area will have a health food store at which many varieties of protein powder are sold. For any of you who do not have access to such a store, here are several sources by mail. Most of these companies have more than one protein powder, and many of them contain high levels of carbohydrate, so ask specifically for the products listed in Chapter 6. This is by no means an exclusive list; go to a health food store or a pharmacy and use the guidelines for a complete protein outlined in Chapter 6 to find one that suits your taste if none of these is available and you don't want to wait for the mail.

MLO Products Company
260 Link Road
Suite A
Suisun, CA 94585
1-800-228-4656

Joe Weider Products
Weider
2677 El Presidio St.
Carson, CA 90810
Toll-free number: 1-800-382-3399 (or 1-800-423-5713 in California)

RDA Products
Lewis Laboratories
Telephone: 1-203-226-7343
Toll-free number: 1-800-243-6020 (Ask for mail-order department)

Sportstar Health and Fitness
P.O. Box 24594
Tempe, AZ 85285-4594
Telephone: 1-602-829-7557
Toll-free number: 1-800-255-7557

General Nutrition Centers Challenge Products
at GNC stores nationwide
National GNC telephone number: 1-800-458-0896

Low-Carbohydrate Recipes and Solka Floc (Crystalline Cellulose)
William Mark Parker
Delicious Low-Carbohydrate Recipes
6055 Primacy Parkway, Suite 401
Memphis, TN 38119
Mr. Parker hopes to have Solka Floc, packaged in small amounts for
individual sale, available soon. At present, it is only sold commercially—
in truckloads. That amount may be slightly more than you will need in
your pantry.

Fatty Acid Supplements
BioSyn has several products that are food-based, don't require
prescriptions, and are very effective. They have a product that produces
the same effects as does Retin-A, another that restores lost hair, and yet
another that lowers cholesterol. These products are in addition to the
superb O-3/O-6 fatty acid supplements. Call or write them for
information; and tell them you read about the products in this book and
they will send you an information packet.

BioSyn
21 Tioga Way
Marblehead, MA 01945
Telephone: 1-617-639-2401
Toll-free number: 1-800-346-2703

Crème Fraîche and Fresh Goat Cheese
Delicious crème fraîche is used in several of our recipes. It is luscious as a
topping as well. During the weight-loss phase, it carries too high a calorie
cost, so save it for maintenance. Used judiciously, it is a fabulous treat.

Kendall Cheese Co.
P.O. Box 686
Atascadero, CA 93423
Telephone: 1-805-466-7252

Konsyl Powder

The manufacturer assures me that pharmaceutical wholesalers all across the country have Konsyl available. Just ask the pharmacist in your area to order the product. The pharmacist can get the name of the wholesaler or distributor in any area by contacting the Boots Pharmaceutical Company in Shreveport, Louisiana, at 1-318-861-8200.

Canola Oil Mayonnaise

I found a manufacturer that makes a good canola oil mayonnaise high in monounsaturated fat. At this time this product cannot be purchased through the mail, but it is in health food stores nationwide. A company representative told me that they would try to assist any readers who might have trouble finding this product by helping them locate a store in their area that carries it. The product is called Spectrum Naturals Canola Mayonnaise.

Spectrum Marketing
133 Copeland Street
Petaluma, CA 94952
1-707-778-8900 (Ask for customer service)

Carbohydrate Content Sources

Food Values of Portions Commonly Used, 14th ed.
revised by Jean A.T. Pennington and Helen Nichols Church
New York: Perennial Library, 1985

Calories and Carbohydrates, 7th rev. ed.
by Barbara Kraus
New York: Signet Books, 1987

The All-in-One Carbohydrate Gram Counter
by Jean Carper
New York: Bantam, 1987

Newsletter

I am preparing a monthly newsletter for my patients that will include new, tested low-carbohydrate recipes and the results of the latest medical research on fats, fatty acid supplementation, and health and dietary matters in general. If you are interested in receiving the newsletter, please send your name and address for subscription information to:

Newsletter
8116 Cantrell Road—Suite C
Little Rock, AR 72207

APPENDIX C

Effective Carbohydrate Content (ECC) of Food

FRUITS

Food Name	Portion	ECC	Carbohydrate	Fiber
Apple juice—frzn	½ cup	14.9	14.9	0.0
Apple juice—canned	½ cup	14.7	15.0	0.3
Apple—raw/peeled	1 item	18.1	21.1	2.9
Apples—dried/uncooked	¼ cup	13.8	16.3	2.5
Apples—raw/unpeeled	1 item	17.6	20.8	3.2
Applesauce—can/unsweet	½ cup	13.2	15.6	2.4
Apricot—raw	1 item	3.3	4.0	0.7
Apricot nectar—canned	½ cup	15.1	15.4	0.3
Apricots—canned/in water	1 cup	10.5	14.3	3.8
Apricots—can/in juice	½ cup	14.0	15.4	1.4
Apricots—canned/syrup	⅓ cup	15.1	15.6	0.5
Apricots—dried/uncooked	¼ cup	13.5	15.5	2.0
Banana—raw	½ item	13.8	15.3	1.5
Blackberries—frzn/unsw	⅔ cup	10.0	14.7	4.7
Blackberries—raw	¾ cup	7.7	14.9	7.2
Blueberries—frzn/unsw	¾ cup	10.7	14.5	3.8
Blueberries—raw	¾ cup	9.1	15.0	5.9
Boysenberries—frzn/unsw	1 cup	9.9	14.6	4.7
Cherries, sour—unsw	¾ cup	12.7	14.3	1.6
Cherries, sour—can/water	⅔ cup	14.6	15.0	0.4
Cherries, sweet—can	½ cup	14.9	15.2	0.3
Cherries, raw sweet	12 items	12.6	13.8	1.2
Cherries, sour—can/syrup	¼ cup	15.2	15.4	0.2
Cherries, sweet—can/water	½ cup	15.1	15.4	0.3
Cranapple juice, lowcal	12 oz	13.2	13.2	0.0
Cranapple juice—canned	⅓ cup	15.3	15.3	0.0
Cranberry juice—bottled	⅓ cup	15.4	15.4	0.0
Cranberry juice, lowcal	10 oz	15.0	15.0	0.0
Cranberry sauce—can/sweet	⅛ cup	15.0	15.5	0.5
Dates—dried/whole	1 item	5.6	6.4	0.8
Elderberries—raw	½ cup	8.3	15.3	7.0
Figs—dried/raw	⅛ cup	13.7	15.4	1.7
Figs—raw	1 item	6.9	10.3	3.5
Fruit cocktail—can/water	¾ cup	14.7	15.9	1.2
Fruit cocktail—can/syrup	½ cup	14.8	15.6	0.8

Food Name	Portion	ECC	Carbohydrate	Fiber
Fruit, mixed—can/syrup	⅓ cup	14.6	15.6	1.0
Fruit, salad—can/water	⅓ cup	11.9	15.6	3.7
Fruit, salad—can/in juice	½ cup	14.8	15.6	0.8
Gooseberries—raw	1 cup	10.1	13.7	3.6
Gooseberries—can/syrup	⅓ cup	13.0	15.3	2.3
Grape juice—canned	⅓ cup	14.7	14.7	0.0
Grape juice—frzn	½ cup	13.6	15.0	1.4
Grapefruit—can/water	⅔ cup	14.1	15.2	1.1
Grapefruit—raw	½ item	8.9	10.1	1.3
Grapefruit juice	⅔ cup	13.9	14.2	0.3
Grapefruit juice (unsw)	⅔ cup	14.3	14.3	0.0
Grapes—raw	½ cup	13.5	14.9	1.4
Grapes—raw/American	1 cup	14.7	16.3	1.6
Guavas, strawberry—raw	15 items	9.1	15.6	6.5
Melon, casaba—raw	1 cup	9.0	11.2	2.2
Melon, honeydew—raw	1 cup	14.1	15.6	1.5
Nectarines—raw	1 item	11.6	14.3	2.7
Orange juice—fresh	½ cup	12.8	13.9	1.1
Orange juice—canned	½ cup	13.9	14.1	0.2
Orange juice—frozen	½ cup	14.0	14.4	0.4
Orange-grapefruit juice	½ cup	14.2	14.2	0.0
Oranges—raw	1 item	12.4	14.9	2.5
Papaya—raw	1 cup	13.8	15.2	1.4
Papaya nectar—canned	½ cup	15.2	15.3	0.1
Passion-fruit juice	⅓ cup	13.9	14.4	0.5
Peach nectar—canned	½ cup	15.3	15.5	0.2
Peaches—dried/uncooked	⅛ cup	13.2	15.4	2.2
Peaches—can/water pack	1 cup	14.3	15.4	1.1
Peaches—raw/whole	1 item	8.3	10.4	2.1
Pear—raw/unpeeled	½ item	12.4	15.3	2.9
Pear nectar—canned	⅓ cup	15.2	15.9	0.7
Pears—can/water	⅔ cup	12.6	16.1	3.5
Pears—can/in juice	½ cup	13.3	15.6	2.3
Pineapple—raw	¾ cup	13.1	15.0	1.9
Pineapple juice—canned	½ cup	14.7	14.8	0.1
Pineapple juice—frzn	½ cup	14.7	14.8	0.1
Pineapple-grapefruit juice	½ cup	15.0	15.0	0.0
Pineapple-orange juice	½ cup	14.5	14.5	0.0
Pineapple—can/in juice	⅓ cup	14.9	15.7	0.8
Plums—can/in juice	⅓ cup	15.3	15.7	0.4
Plums—can/water	⅔ cup	15.5	16.2	0.7
Plums—raw/prune-type	3 items	16.2	18.0	1.8
Pomegranate—raw	½ item	14.6	15.2	0.6
Prune juice—canned	⅓ cup	14.6	14.7	0.1
Prunes—canned/syrup	¼ cup	13.8	15.9	2.1
Prunes—dried/uncooked	⅛ cup	14.0	15.7	1.7

Food Name	Portion	ECC	Carbohydrate	Fiber
Pummelo—raw/sections	¾ cup	13.9	15.5	1.6
Raisins—seedless	⅛ cup	14.2	15.9	1.7
Raspberries—frzn/sweet	¼ cup	12.7	15.3	2.6
Raspberries—raw	1 cup	8.5	13.9	5.4
Rhubarb—cooked w/sugar	⅛ cup	14.5	15.3	0.8
Rhubarb—frzn/cooked w/sugar	¼ cup	15.1	16.1	1.0
Strawberries—whole/raw	1 cup	7.8	11.2	3.4
Strawberries—frzn/unsweet	1 cup	9.0	12.6	3.6
Tangerine juice—fresh	½ cup	13.8	14.2	0.4
Tangerines—raw	½ item	12.5	15.2	2.7
Tangerines—can/in juice	⅔ cup	14.5	15.5	1.0
Tangerines—can/lt. syrup	⅓ cup	15.5	16.0	0.5
Watermelon—raw	1 cup	10.7	11.0	0.3

VEGETABLES

Food Name	Portion	ECC	Carbohydrate	Fiber
Artichokes—boiled	1 item	8.6	12.6	4.1
Asparagus—raw/boiled	⅔ cup	3.6	5.0	1.4
Beans, green or wax—frzn/boil	¾ cup	4.7	6.4	1.7
Beans, green—canned	1 cup	4.7	6.6	1.9
Beans, green—raw/boiled	⅔ cup	4.9	6.3	1.4
Beans, wax—raw/boiled	⅔ cup	4.9	6.3	1.4
Beets—canned/sliced	¾ cup	6.0	8.2	2.2
Broccoli—frzn/boiled	½ cup	1.4	5.4	4.0
Broccoli—raw	1 cup	1.4	4.3	3.0
Broccoli—raw/boiled	1 cup	2.1	8.0	5.9
Brussels sprouts—frzn/boiled	½ cup	3.7	5.6	1.9
Brussels sprouts—raw/boiled	½ cup	4.2	6.3	2.1
Cabbage, red—raw/shredded	1 cup	2.5	4.2	1.7
Cabbage—boiled	1 cup	2.7	6.4	3.7
Cabbage—raw/shredded	1 cup	2.7	4.2	1.5
Carrot—raw/whole	1 item	4.8	6.6	1.8
Carrots—boiled/sliced	1 cup	12.6	19.5	6.9
Cauliflower—frzn/boiled	1 cup	3.9	7.4	3.6
Cauliflower—raw/boiled	1 cup	3.3	5.4	2.1
Cauliflower—raw/chopped	1 cup	2.1	4.6	2.5
Celery—raw/stalk	5 items	4.9	6.8	1.9
Chard, Swiss—boiled	¾ cup	2.9	5.8	2.9
Chard, Swiss—raw	5 cups	3.5	6.2	2.7
Cucumber—raw/sliced	2 cups	3.1	6.0	2.9
Eggplant—boiled	1 cup	3.9	6.8	2.9
Greens, beet—boiled	1 cup	3.6	8.3	4.7
Greens, chicory—raw/chopped	1 cup	4.1	8.4	4.4
Greens, collard—boiled	1 cup	3.0	5.2	2.2

Food Name	Portion	ECC	Carbohydrate	Fiber
Greens, collard—frzn/boiled	1 cup	6.4	11.2	4.8
Greens, dandelion—boiled	1 cup	2.8	7.2	4.4
Greens, mustard—boiled	1 cup	0.3	3.1	2.8
Greens, turnip—raw/boiled	1 cup	3.0	6.1	3.1
Juice, carrot—canned	½ cup	9.6	13.0	3.4
Juice, tomato—canned	⅔ cup	5.0	6.9	1.9
Juice, V-8 vegetable	½ cup	3.8	5.3	1.5
Juice, vegetable—canned	⅔ cup	5.3	7.0	1.7
Kale—frzn/boiled	1 cup	2.9	6.5	3.6
Kale—raw/boiled	1 cup	3.0	7.4	4.4
Leeks—boiled	1 item	6.3	9.3	3.1
Lentils—cooked/whole	⅓ cup	10.0	13.4	3.4
Lettuce—shredded	2 cups	1.2	2.4	1.2
Mushrooms—boiled	9 items	3.7	5.7	2.0
Mushrooms—raw/chopped	1 cup	2.0	3.4	1.3
Okra—raw/boiled	½ cup	5.3	6.4	1.1
Onion, mature—boiled	½ cup	5.6	6.4	0.8
Parsnips—sliced/boiled	½ cup	13.1	17.4	4.3
Peas & carrots—frzn/boiled	1 cup	8.6	15.3	6.7
Peas, green—canned	⅔ cup	8.8	13.1	4.3
Peas, podded—raw	1 cup	2.9	10.4	7.5
Peppers, sweet—raw	1 item	3.0	4.1	1.1
Radishes—raw/sliced	1 cup	2.4	6.4	4.0
Rutabagas—boiled	½ cup	5.2	6.4	1.2
Spinach—boiled	⅔ cup	2.3	4.6	2.3
Spinach—frzn/boiled	½ cup	3.2	5.3	2.1
Squash, acorn—baked	⅔ cup	16.0	18.7	2.7
Squash, butternut—baked	¾ cup	15.7	18.7	3.0
Squash, summer—boiled	1 cup	4.6	7.8	3.2
Squash, winter—baked	1 cup	13.1	16.3	3.2
Squash, zucchini—frzn/boiled	¾ cup	3.6	6.0	2.4
Squash, zucchini—raw/boiled	1 cup	4.7	7.0	2.3
Tomato—canned/whole	⅔ cup	4.9	6.1	1.2
Tomato—raw	1 item	3.0	5.0	2.0
Tomato—raw/boiled	½ cup	5.5	6.3	0.8
Turnips—boiled/diced	1 cup	5.6	7.6	2.0
Vegetables, mixed—frzn/boiled	⅔ cup	13.1	15.9	2.8

BREADS AND SNACK FOODS

Food Name	Portion	ECC	Carbohydrate	Fiber
Bagel	1 item	27.0	27.4	0.4
Bread, Colonial light	1 slice	6.0	9.0	3.0
Bread, Wonder light	1 slice	7.0	10.0	3.0
Bread, pumpernickel	1 slice	12.6	13.6	1.0
Bread, raisin	1 slice	13.1	13.7	0.6
Granola	¼ cup	12.3	13.2	0.9
Peanut butter, smooth	2 tbsp	2.5	5.0	2.5
Peanuts, oil-roasted	1 oz	2.2	5.0	2.8
Popcorn, popped—plain	2 cups	8.8	9.6	0.8
Pork rinds—plain	2 cups	0.0	0.0	0.0
Potato chips	15 items	15.6	16.0	0.4

Please note that even in these cases, there are few carbohydrate bargains in the bread, cereal, and snack categories.

SOURCE: Database in auto-Nutritionist III software program developed by N² N-Squared Computing, 5318 Forest Ridge Road, Silverton, OR 97381

Bibliographic Notes

Chapter 1
"Mortality: Obesity Increases the Risk for Heart Disease, Cancer and Diabetes." *Obesity International Newsletter* 1, no. 10 (November 1987).

"Overweight Adults in the United States," ADVANCEDATA, from Vital and Health Statistics of the National Center for Health Statistics, U.S. Department of Health, Education and Welfare, DHEW Publication No. 79–1250 (August 30, 1979).

Chapter 2
Bistrian, Bruce. "Clinical Use of a Protein-Sparing Modified Fast." *Journal of the American Medical Association* 240, no. 21 (November 17, 1978).

Bistrian, B. R., et al. "Nitrogen Metabolism and Insulin Requirements in Obese Diabetic Adults." *Diabetes* 25, no. 6 (1976).

Blackburn, G. L., et al. "Peripheral Intravenous Feeding with Isotonic Amino Acid Solutions." *American Journal of Surgery* 125 (April 1973).

———. "Role of a Protein-Sparing Modified Fast in a Comprehensive Weight Reduction Program." *Recent Advances in Obesity Research*. London: Newman, 1974.

Brown, Jerry M., et al. "Cardiac Complications of Protein-Sparing Modified Fasting." *Journal of the American Medical Association* 240, no. 2 (July 14, 1978).

Genuth, Saul, "Supplemented Fasting in the Treatment of Obesity and Diabetes." *American Journal of Clinical Nutrition* 32 (December 1979).

Genuth, Saul, et al. "Weight Reduction in Obesity by Outpatient Semi-starvation." *Journal of the American Medical Association* 230, no. 7 (November 18, 1974).

————. "Supplemented Fasting in the Treatment of Obesity." *Recent Advances in Obesity Research—II* London: John Libbey & Company Ltd.: 370–378.

Henry, R. R., et al. "Metabolic Consequences of Very-Low-Calorie Diet Therapy in Obese Non-Insulin-Dependent Diabetic and Nondiabetic Subjects." *Diabetes* 35 (February 1986).

Hoffer, Leonard, J., et al. "Metabolic Effects of Very Low Calorie Weight Reduction Diets." *American Journal for Clinical Investigations* 73 (March 1984).

Kirschner, Marvin, et al. "Supplemented Starvation: A Successful Method for Control of Major Obesity." *Journal of the Medical Society of New Jersey* 76, no. 3 (March 1979).

Linet, O. I., et al. "Absence of Cardiac Arrhythmias During a Very-Low-Calorie Diet with High Biological Quality Protein." *International Journal of Obesity* 7 (1983).

"Liquid Protein Mayhem." Editorial, *Journal of the American Medical Association* 240, no. 2 (July 14, 1978).

Palgi, Aviva, et al. "Multidisciplinary Treatment of Obesity with a Protein-Sparing Modified Fast Results in 668 Outpatients." *American Journal of Public Health* 75, no. 10 (October 1985).

Singh, Bramah N., et al. "Liquid Protein Diets and *Torsade de Pointes*." *Journal of the American Medical Association* 240, no. 2 (July 14, 1978).

Van Gaal, Luc, et al. "Anthropometric and Calorimetric Evidence for the Protein-Sparing Effects of a New Protein Supplemented Low Calorie Preparation." *Endocrinology, Metabolism, and Nutrition* 41 (1985).

Vertes, Victor, et al. "Supplemented Fasting as a Large-Scale Outpatient Program." *Journal of the American Medical Association* 238, no. 20 (November 14, 1977).

Wadden, Thomas, et al. "Very Low Calorie Diets: Their Efficacy, Safety and Future." *Annals of Internal Medicine*, 99 (1983).

Winterer, Joerg, et al. "Whole Body Protein Turnover, Studied with N-Glycine and Muscle Protein Breakdown in Mildly Obese Subjects During a Protein-Sparing Diet and a Brief Total Fast." *Metabolism* 29, no. 6 (June 1980).

Chapter 3
Crapo, Phyllis A., et al. "Comparison of Serum Glucose, Insulin, and Glucagen Responses to Different Types of Complex Carbohydrate in Noninsulin-Dependent Diabetic Patients." *American Journal of Clinical Nutrition* 34 (February 1981): 184–190.

Cunningham, John. *Introduction to Nutritional Physiology*. Philadelphia: George F. Stickley Company, 1983.

Davenport, Horace W. *Physiology of the Digestive Tract*. 5th ed. Chicago: Year Book Medical Publishers, Inc., 1982.

Jenkins, David J. A., et al. "Glycemic Index of Foods: A Physiological Basis of Carbohydrate Exchange." *American Journal of Clinical Nutrition* 34 (March 1981): 362–366.

―――. "The Glycemic Index of Foods Tested in Diabetic Patients: A New Basis of Carbohydrate Exchange Favoring the Use of Legumes." *Diabetologia* 24 (1983): 257–264.

Miles, Carolyn, et al. "Effect of Dietary Fiber on the Metabolizable Energy of Human Diets." *American Institute of Nutrition* (1988).

National Academy of Sciences. *Recommended Dietary Allowances*. 9th ed. Washington, D.C.: National Academy Press (1980).

Shils, Maurice, and V. Young, eds. *Modern Nutrition in Health and Disease*. 7th ed. Philadelphia: Lea & Febiger, 1988.

Sirtori, Cesare R., et al. "Controlled Evaluation of Fat Intake in the Mediterranean Diet: Comparative Activities of Olive Oil and Corn Oil on Plasma Lipids and Platelets in High-Risk Patients." *American Journal of Clinical Nutrition* 44 (1986): 635–642.

Stryer, Lubert. *Biochemistry*. 3rd ed. New York: W. H. Freeman and Company, 1988.

Young, V. R., and P. Pellett. "Protein Intake and Requirements with Reference to Diet and Health." *American Journal of Clinical Nutrition* 45 (1987): 1323–1343.

Chapter 4

Fisher, A. Garth. *The Complete Book of Physical Fitness.* Salt Lake City: Brigham University Press, 1979.

Forbes, G. B., and S. L. Welle. "Lean Body Mass in Obesity." *International Journal of Obesity* 7 (1983): 99–107.

Ganong, William F. *Review of Medical Physiology.* 13th ed. Norwalk, Connecticut: Appleton & Lange, 1987.

Lukaski, Henry C., et al. "Validation of Tetrapolar Bioelectrical Impedance Method to Assess Human Body Composition." *Journal of Applied Physiology* 60, no. 4 (1986): 1327–1332.

Penrose, K. W., et al. "Generalized Body Composition Prediction Equation for Men Using Simple Measurement Techniques." *Medicine and Science in Sports and Exercise* 17, no. 2 (1985).

Remington, Dennis, et al. *How to Lower Your Fat Thermostat.* Provo, Utah: Vitality House International, Inc., 1983.

Stryer, Lubert. *Biochemistry.* 3rd ed. New York: W. H. Freeman and Company, 1988.

Chapter 5

Brown, Marilyn R., et al. "A High Protein, Low Calorie Liquid Diet in the Treatment of Very Obese Adolescents: Long-Term Effect on Lean Body Mass." *American Journal of Clinical Nutrition* 38, no. 1 (July 1983).

Chapter 6

Amatruda, John M., et al. "Vigorous Supplementation of a Hypocaloric Diet Prevents Cardiac Arrhythmias and Mineral Depletion." *American Journal of Medicine* 74 (June 1983).

Chapter 8

Jones, D. Yvonne, et al. "Influence of Caloric Contribution and Saturation of Dietary Fat on Plasma Lipids in Premenopausal Women." *American Journal of Clinical Nutrition* 45 (1987): 1451–6.

Taylor, Elizabeth. *Elizabeth Takes Off.* New York: G. P. Putnam's Sons, 1987.

Yudkin, John. "Low Carbohydrate Diet in Treatment of Obesity." *Postgraduate Medicine* 51, no. 5 (1972).

Chapter 9

LaBell, Fran. "Powdered Cellulose Adds Texture, High Fiber to Reduced Calorie Foods." *Food Processing* (July 1986).

Miller, William B. "Seeing the 'Light,' Cellulose in Reduced-Calorie Baked Goods." *Baker's Digest* (July 10, 1986).

Chapter 10

Brussaard, Jantine H., et al. "Serum Lipoproteins of Healthy Persons Fed a Low-Fat Diet or a Polyunsaturated Fat Diet for Three Months." *Atherosclerosis* 42 (1982): 205–219.

Cade, J. E., et al. "Diet and Inequalities in Health in Three English Towns." *British Medical Journal* 296 (May 14, 1988).

"Cardiovascular Effects of n-3 Fatty Acids." Editorial, *New England Journal of Medicine* 319, no. 9 (September 1, 1988).

Coulston, Ann M., et al. "Plasma Glucose, Insulin and Lipid Responses to High-Carbohydrate Low-Fat Diets in Normal Humans." *Metabolism* 32, no. 1 (January 1983).

Eaton, S. Boyd, and M. Konner. "Paleolithic Nutrition." *New England Journal of Medicine* 312, no. 5 (January 31, 1985).

"Fish Oil." Editorial, *The Lancet* (May 14, 1980).

Grundy, Scott M. "Comparison of Monounsaturated Fatty Acids and Carbohydrates for Lowering Plasma Cholesterol." *New England Journal of Medicine* 314, no. 12 (March 20, 1986).

International Collaborative Study Group. "Metabolic Epidemiology of Plasma Cholesterol." *The Lancet* (November 1, 1986).

Kernoff, P.B.A., et al. "Anti-Thrombotic Potential of Dihomo Gamma Linolenic Acid." *British Medical Journal II* (1977).

Kromhout, D., et al. "The Inverse Relation Between Fish Consumption and 20-Year Mortality from Coronary Heart Disease." *New England Journal of Medicine* 312 (1985).

Leaf, Alexander, and P. Weber. "Cardiovascular Effects of n-3 Fatty Acids." *New England Journal of Medicine* 318, no. 9 (March 3, 1988).

Lee, T. H., et al. "Effect of Dietary Enrichment with Eicosapentaenoic and Docosahexaenoic Acids on In Vitro Neutrophil and Monocyte Leukotriene Generation and Neutrophil Function." *New England Journal of Medicine* 312 (1985).

Mattson, Fred H., and S. Grundy. "Comparison of Effects of Dietary Saturated, Monounsaturated, and Polyunsaturated Fatty Acids on Plasma Lipids and Lipoproteins in Man." *Journal of Lipid Research* 26 (1985).

Manninen, V., et al. "Lipid Alterations and Decline in the Incidence of Coronary Heart Disease in the Helsinki Heart Study." *Journal of the American Medical Association* 260, no. 5 (August 5, 1988).

Mensink, Ronald, and M. Katan. "Effect of Monounsaturated Fatty Acids versus Complex Carbohydrates on High-Density Lipoproteins in Healthy Men and Women." *The Lancet* (January 17, 1987).

Miettinen, Tatu A. "Dietary Fiber and Lipids." *American Journal of Clinical Nutrition* 45 (1987).

Nauss, Kathleen M., et al. "Dietary Fat and Fiber: Relationship to Caloric Intake, Body Growth, and Colon Tumorigenesis." *American Journal of Clinical Nutrition* 45 (1987).

Phillipson, B. E., et al. "Reduction of Plasma Lipids, Lipoproteins, and Apoproteins by Dietary Fish Oils in Patients with Hypertriglyceridemia." *New England Journal of Medicine* 312 (1985).

Riccardi, G., et al. "Separate Influence of Dietary Carbohydrate and Fiber on the Metabolic Control of Diabetes." *Diabetologia* 26 (1984).

Ross, Russell. "The Pathogenesis of Atherosclerosis—An Update." *New England Journal of Medicine* 314, no. 8 (February 20, 1986).

Schatzkin, Arthur, et al. "Serum Cholesterol and Cancer in the NHanes I Epidemiologic Follow-up Study." *The Lancet* (August 8, 1987).

von Schacky, et al. "Long-Term Effects of Dietary Marine Omega 3 Fatty Acids upon Plasma and Cellular Lipids, Platelet Function, and Eicosanoid Formation in Humans." *Journal of Clinical Investigation* 76 (1985).

Yetiv, Jack Z. "Clinical Applications of Fish Oils." *Journal of the American Medical Association* 260, no. 5 (August 5, 1988).

Ziboh, V. A., et al. "Effects of Dietary Supplementation of Fish Oil on Neutrophil and Epidermal Fatty Acids. Modulation of Clinical Course of Psoriatic Subjects." *Archives of Dermatology* 122 (1986).

Chapter 11

Andersen, E., et al. "Effects of a High-Protein and Low-Fat Diet vs. a Low-Protein and High-Fat Diet on Blood Glucose, Serum Lipoproteins, and Cholesterol Metabolism in Noninsulin Dependent Diabetics." *American Journal of Clinical Nutrition* 45 (1987).

Bonanome, Andrea, and S. Grundy. "Effect of Dietary Stearic Acid on Plasma Cholesterol and Lipoprotein Levels." *New England Journal of Medicine* 318, no. 19 (May 12, 1988).

Coulston, Ann M., et al. "Deleterious Metabolic Effects of High-Carbohydrate, Sucrose-Containing Diets in Patients with Noninsulin-Dependent Diabetes Mellitus." *American Journal of Medicine* 82 (February 1987).

"Dietary Saturated Fatty Acids and Blood Cholesterol." Editorial, *New England Journal of Medicine* 318, no. 19 (May 12, 1988).

"Dietary Therapy for Noninsulin-Dependent Diabetes Mellitus." Editorial, *New England Journal of Medicine* 319, no. 13 (September 29, 1988).

Fuh, M. M-T., et al. "Abnormalities of Carbohydrate and Lipid Metabolism in Patients with Hypertension." *Archives of Internal Medicine* 147 (June 1987).

Garg, Abhimanyu, et al. "Comparison of a High-Carbohydrate Diet with a High-Monounsaturated-Fat Diet in Patients with Noninsulin-Dependent Diabetes Mellitus." *New England Journal of Medicine* 319, no. 13 (September 29, 1988).

Newbold, H. L. "Reducing the Serum Cholesterol Level with a Diet High in Animal Fat." *Southern Medical Journal* 81, no. 1 (January 1988).

Parillo, Mario, et al. "Effect of a Low-Fat Diet on Carbohydrate Metabolism in Patients with Hypertension." *Hypertension* 11, no. 3 (March 1988).

Reaven, G. M. "How High the Carbohydrate?" *Diabetologia* 19 (1980).

Rudney, Harry, and R. Sexton. "Regulation of Cholesterol Biosynthesis." *Annual Review of Nutrition* 6 (1986).

Wolf, Richard N., and S. Grundy. "Influence of Exchanging Carbohydrate for Saturated Fatty Acids on Plasma Lipids and Lipoproteins in Men." *Journal of Nutrition* 113 (1983).

Chapter 13
Balady, G. J., et al. "Comparison of Determinants of Myocardial Oxygen Consumption During Arm and Leg Exercises in Normal Persons." *American Journal of Cardiology* 57 (1986).

Bar-Shlomo, B.-Z., et al. "Left Ventricular Function in Trained and Untrained Healthy Subjects." *Circulation* 65 (1982).

Blair, S. N., et al. "Physical Fitness and Incidence of Hypertension in Healthy Normotensive Men and Women." *Journal of the American Medical Association* 252 (1984).

Cailliet, Rene, and Leonard Gross. *The Rejuvenation Strategy*. New York, Doubleday and Company, 1987.

Eichner, E. R. "Exercise and Heart Disease: Epidemiology of the 'Exercise Hypothesis,' " *American Journal of Medicine* 75 (1983).

Hammond, H. K., and V. F. Froelicher. "Normal and Abnormal Heart Rate Responses to Exercise." *Progress in Cardiovascular Disease* 27 (1985).

Hollosky, J. Q., et al. "Physiological Consequences of the Biochemical Adaptations to Endurance Exercise." *Annals of the New York Academy of Sciences* 301 (1977).

Martin, B. J. and J. M. Stager. "Ventilatory Endurance in Athletes and Nonathletes." *Medical Science and Sports Exercise* 13 (1981).

Rigotti, N. A., et al. "Exercise and Coronary Heart Disease." *Annual Review of Medicine* 34 (1983).

Saltin, B. "Hemodynamic Adaptations to Exercise." *American Journal of Cardiology* 55 (1985).

Simon, H. B., and S. R. Levisohn. *The Athlete Within: A Personal Guide to Total Fitness*. Boston: Little, Brown and Company, 1987.

Wasserman, K. "Breathing During Exercise." *New England Journal of Medicine* 298 (1978).

Wilcox, R. G., et al. "Is Exercise Good for High Blood Pressure?" *British Medical Journal* 285 (1982).

Chapter 14
Glasser, William. *Take Effective Control of Your Life*. New York, Harper & Row, 1984.

Index

Recipe Index